The Survivor's N

A DISASTER SURVIVAL GUIDE

By Cass Igram, D.O.

Dedication: To all those who have endured the crises of natural disasters, especially to those who have lost loved ones.

Disclaimer: The information contained in this book is not meant for the diagnosis or treatment of disease. Individuals who suffer from serious medical conditions must consult their physicians before undergoing any change in treatment or attempting additional treatment.

Revised Edition

ISBN: 0911119-44-2

Knowledge House Publishers

Printed by Cedar Graphics
311 Parsons Drive
Hiawatha, Iowa 52233-1458

For ordering information call 1-800-243-5242

Table of Contents

Introduction

Today, we live in a highly dangerous and incredibly toxic world. Earthquakes, floods, volcanoes, tidal waves, smog, mass transport accidents, radiation leakages and toxic chemical spills torment the earth.

Since the inception of humankind, there have always existed inherent dangers to its existence. History is replete with examples of natural disasters which have crippled civilizations and, in some instances, destroyed them. However, modern man has complicated this by producing additional dangers. Now the human race is faced with the added burden of man-made or, more descriptively, "un-natural" disasters.

In this modern era natural disasters are the least of our problems. The human race has fouled the universe, and most of the blame lies on the industrialized world, specifically the United States, Canada, Britain, France, Germany, Japan and Russia. No part of this earth remains unscathed from man's caustic pollutants. Incredible as it may seem, most of the fresh water supplies are contaminated. Some lakes and rivers are so defiled that swimming in them is prohibited and the fish within them cannot be consumed. Even the oceans are polluted. The air over much of the earth is foul. The land is contaminated by industrial and agricultural chemicals. Certain regions of the earth, notably toxic dumps, are so dangerous that they may be entered only at the risk of serious illness or death.

To many, this may seem a pessimistic view. However, Chernobyl, Bhopal, Love Canal, Three Mile Island and the near daily event in the U.S.A. of major toxic chemical spills/releases prove that today's world is incredibly dangerous and that much of this danger is man-made.

Industrialists, politicians and scientists have gone to great lengths to assure the American public that the toxicity of synthetic chemicals to the environment and to animal, plant and human life is minimal. What toxicity they do admit is regarded as a necessary consequence of modernization and "human progress." The chemists and industrialists, as well as other supporters of synthetics, should take note that all of the above-mentioned disasters were caused by the chemicals they create. Are these chemicals so crucial that all the wonderment and beauty the earth beholds must be held at risk? Are they worth the systematic destruction of the plant and animal kingdom? Must man continue to sterilize the earth with toxic chemicals and nuclear radiation? This is madness. The "We can't live without them" argument is out of vogue. On the contrary, evidence is accumulating that man won't be able to inhabit this planet much longer unless the use of toxic chemicals is curtailed.

The nuclear age was a waste, literally. As it turns out, Russia never was and probably never will be a threat to U.S. soil. All those nuclear armaments that were, and still are, being tested -- what for?

Chernobyl was the most destructive of the nuclear plant accidents. Yet, there have been hundreds of "mini-Chernobyls," accidents which have spewed untold billions of particles of radioactive contaminants. The industrial powers have irradiated every living creature on this earth. The consequences will ultimately be devastating. Perhaps most frightening will be the rise in the incidence of certain types of cancers, which will reach such high levels that they will soon be regarded as massive epidemics. Do not be shocked if this happens, and do not be surprised if the authorities claim the cause to be "unknown." In fact, it is already happening. People must take steps to protect our bodies from the unrelenting release of destructive radioactive chemicals to which all Americans are currently being exposed. The least that can be done is to consume those nutrients which impede and/or reverse the toxicity of radioactive chemicals.

Recent reports (March, 1992) indicate that Russia alone contributed 270 nuclear plant accidents to the world burden of radiation. Further, the ill effects of Chernobyl are lingering and not just in Russia. A recent (March, 1992) New York times report notes that scientists in Russia have found "widespread degradation" of the health of tens of thousands of people who were in the path of Chernobyl's fallout.

The atmosphere is polluted. Must we continue to pollute it? The ground water is laced with thousands of noxious contaminants. Must we continue to turn our precious fresh water supplies into carcinogenic chemical soups? Our soils are defiled by countless thousands of noxious compounds. Must we continue to desecrate the land wherein our food is grown and upon which our homes reside? How much more toxic can the earth become?

In July, 1991, the *Los Angeles Times* reported that, "A foul-smelling plume of poisonous metam-sodium...killed all aquatic life along a 45-mile stretch of the Sacramento River." Forty-five miles of death, decimation and destruction. "Sterilized" was the term used by one reporter describing the river bed. "Extinct" was the description given by a biologist examining the destruction. It seems that there are no words which would thoroughly describe the scope of the damage from this tragedy.

This disaster was due to a train derailment in an isolated region of Northern California. Only one tanker car was punctured. In the event of a massive earthquake, hundreds of such spills could theoretically occur. This is not pessimism. It is a fact of life -- or death.

When the earthquake strikes and toxic spills or nuclear radiation leakages occur, the chemists, industrialists, politicians and economists will be nowhere to be found. They will be running for their lives like the rest of us. They, and thousands of others, will be suffering as a consequence of ill-conceived economic, industrial and political strategies.

Nuclear power has been acclaimed as a necessary evil. The same has been said by the makers of pesticides, herbicides, fumigants, dioxins and PCBs. The argument for the necessity of these chemicals is questionable. The fact that they are evil is beyond doubt. Is it not evil that thousands of children in Russia are dying of cancer as a result of the Chernobyl meltdown? Breast tumors are being found in children eight and nine years old. An entire segment of this earth, hundreds of square miles, was left uninhabitable. More recently, a significant nuclear accident occurred here in the United States. This report buried in the back pages of the newspaper stated that 50,000 gallons of radioactive water were "accidentally released" from a nuclear plant in South Carolina. Make no mistake about it, that is a significant amount of radioactive waste. The day after this toxic spill, a report was issued that the plant had to release radioactive steam, "in order to investigate the cause of the spill." This type of noxious radioactive release was described as "not uncommon" from nuclear power plants. The official word was that neither the radioactive water nor steam pose any threat to human life. This is nonsense.

Is it not evil that a catastrophe of this proportion can happen, and then the entire issue of toxicity is "washed over." "Oh, but we do not want to alarm the public," some authorities might claim. Since when did propaganda and cover-up help anyone? The American public would much rather know the truth. Is it not evil that the finest natural trout fishery in Northern California -- one that took decades to cultivate -- was destroyed in a short 24 hours by a fumigant the world could have lived without? Is it not an evil tragedy beyond comprehension that thousands of residents of Bhopal, India, were killed in a most gruesome, violent manner by the release of hydrogen cyanide from an insecticide plant?

The human race has lived adequately for thousands of years without the use of pesticides and/or similar noxious chemicals. Numerous societies successfully cultivated crops similar to those grown today without so much as a drop of pesticide. The earth was clean then. Unfortunately, thanks to pesticides, herbicides, fungicides and other toxic chemicals, the same cannot be said today.

A massive earthquake in California could theoretically result in hundreds of toxic chemical releases. Chemical spills occur daily in California and also across the remainder of the United States, without any provocation from Nature. The July 13th, 1991, spill in the pristine wilderness of Northern California near the town of Dunsmuir has brought to the fore the potential for massive toxic chemical contamination in earthquake zones. Within two weeks there was another massive spill. Again the result of a train derailment; this one occurred in a heavily populated seaside community west of Los Angeles. The chemical was hydrazine, an extremely toxic component of jet and rocket fuel. Concerns of toxicity to humans was so great that a major highway remained closed for nearly a week. There were a total of seven major chemical spills in California in July of 1991 alone.

It is horrifying enough to lose your home and to be stranded as a result of an earthquake. The nightmare of being chased by a toxic cloud is unimaginable, but it can happen to anyone. The toxic compounds may not be located near your home. However, what if a train or truck passes by carrying noxious chemicals such as nuclear wastes, chlorine or bromine gas, liquid oxygen, propane, diesel fuel, propellants, pesticides, herbicides or petrochemicals? These trucks and tanker cars are on the road and rail 24 hours a day every day of the year. Millions of tons of these chemicals are transported in this country every day. In the event of a chemical spill, explosion or gaseous release, neighborhoods could become uninhabitable in a very short time. Nuclear wastes have been spilled in the United States from trucks and tanker cars numerous times; rarely do we hear about it.

Earthquakes are serious business. The people living in San Francisco, Santa Cruz, Watsonville and Mexico City know how devastating they can be. It takes years to repair the damage, and some damage can never be repaired.

Evidence exists that earthquakes have destroyed entire civilizations. Such massive damage is conceivable in California, despite quake-resistant buildings and other preventive measures. If the earthquake is powerful enough, any building could be damaged or destroyed. Entire cities could be reduced to rubble. It just happened in Ferndale, California (April 25, 1992).

The 1992 quakes have arrived and are likely to continue arriving. The warnings have been frequent; the implications are ominous. First it was Turkey, then Southern California, and then, a day later, Southern China. In little more than 48 hours after China's rumblers, the far north of California was bashed by a powerful quake, which caused extensive structural damage and over 50 injuries. The number of injuries were probably limited by the fact that the region is sparsely populated. However, damage within the towns affected was so extensive that a state of emergency was declared. "A major earthquake...knocked people to the ground in Northern California", so reported AP wire news (April 26, 1992), "causing fires and shaking houses off their foundations." This is probably only the beginning; there is every evidence that the big one(s) will strike the earth at any moment. Even if it doesn't happen in 1992, it is just a matter of time.

Even if the big earthquake isn't as destructive as was previously described it is still wise to develop skills in disaster survival. This knowledge would also prove useful during other natural disasters such as tornadoes, hurricanes and floods. Learning how to self-medicate is easier than many people think. When there are no doctors or hospitals available, what choice do people have? Much of our population is entirely dependent upon the medical profession for servicing their health needs. To these individuals, the idea of taking charge of one's health may seem foreign and frightening. If this applies to you, then this book is what you need.

The treatments outlined herein are both easy to apply and safe to use. Even young children can master them. Plus, the knowledge may prove useful in everyday life. The Nutritional Pharmacy provides remedies for home care of colds and flu and for the prevention of sickness when traveling, especially across the borders and overseas. Additionally, it may be utilized as a medicine kit for outdoor activities such as fishing, hiking, backpacking and camping. Most of all, the knowledge contained in this book prepares people for catastrophes which could never be predicted or anticipated. Who would have imagined or anticipated Chernobyl, Bhopal, the Mount St. Helens eruption, Mount Pintatubo, the 1989 Armenian earthquake, the 1989 San Francisco earthquake, the 1991 Oakland fire or the 1992 Guadalajara sewer-line explosion? No longer are the thousands of individuals who suffered through these tragedies deceived by the "it could never happen to me" syndrome. It is likely that they would advise the more fortunate of us who have not suffered to alter our way of thinking and prepare for potential catastrophes *as if they were to happen tomorrow.*

Chapter 1 It Could Happen at Any Time

The Ring of Fire is on fire. For those who are unfamiliar with this term, the Ring describes the highly active geological region on the earth corresponding to the 32nd parallel. This region is located in the Pacific Ocean and includes the land masses bordering it such as Mexico, Alaska and California.

The terminology "Ring of Fire" is self-explanatory: fire represents heat from the earth. The expressions of this heat include hot water springs or geysers, hot air and molten rock (or lava). Thus, the Ring of Fire is a region of intense volcanic and geological activity.

Over the past decade there has been a significant increase in volcanic activity throughout the Ring of Fire. The example most obvious to Americans is the Mount St. Helens eruption of 1980. This volcano is still active. More recently, in June of 1991, a volcano in the Philippines, Mt. Pintatubo, underwent a massive eruption and is still highly active. This volcano had been dormant for over six centuries. In Japan, numerous volcanoes are currently active to the degree that they pose significant threats to the population. A significant potential for volcanic eruptions exists in South America as well, which is also part of the Ring of Fire.

The Pacific Islands are included in the Ring. Many of these are nothing more than the remnants of ancient volcanoes which have surfaced in the oceans. The Hawaiian Islands are the most obvious example. These islands too are areas of intense geological activity.

In January of 1992 Mount Etna in Sicily spewed untold tons of molten rock toward major cities in that island country. This major volcanic eruption threatened and continues to threaten the lives and property of thousands of people.

Even so, it is not the volcanoes that we in the West are most concerned about. It is that potentially cataclysmic geological event associated with increased seismic activity: earthquake.

Earthquakes can be understood by reviewing simple laws of physics. Anything that is heated will expand. Water expands by turning into steam. Metal expands by becoming longer. When the earth becomes excessively hot, according to the laws of physics, it too must expand. Sometimes it releases the excessive heat through increased volcanic activity or through the release of hot air or hot water, as in geysers. At other times the heat builds up to the point that the earth's crust expands and shifts, and that is when earthquakes are likely to occur.

Active volcanoes are a warning that there is a significant increase in the temperature of the earth's crust. They are a sign that increased seismic activity is imminent. They represent a solid clue that major earthquakes are on the way, and soon.

In fact, such earthquakes are occurring now. Three major and several minor quakes have recently hit California. Significant earthquakes have occurred in Oregon and Alaska. Toronto, Canada was struck by one, as was Pennsylvania. Even the Midwest is not immune. The New Madrid fault is currently active. An earthquake recently struck Missouri and Arkansas, an unusual event for those regions, and structural damage to buildings was reported. All of this geological activity occurred in 1991 and 1992.

In August 1991, the most recent Japanese volcanic eruptions caused over 250 earthquakes, tremors and after-shocks. Numerous off-shore tremblers are happening near the shores of Japan, Alaska and California. More recently, in April, 1992, Southern China was rocked by earthquakes measuring nearly 7.0 on the Richter scale.

The seismic activity is moving towards the United States.

First it was the Philippines; then it was Japan; next it will be us. There is every evidence that the big one(s) is/are on the way, especially in California. Perhaps most alarming is the research of two California geologists: Sam Clark and Gary Carver. For years they have studied the so-called Cascadia quake zone located in Northern California. As was recently reported on AP/UPI wire and CNN news, they see significant evidence that the big one is coming. In their words, it will strike "at any time."

In fact, just as this book is going to press the West coast received a critical warning; a quake measuring 6.1 on the Richter scale struck Southern California. The epicenter for this quake was some 100 miles east of Los Angeles. Structural damage to buildings was reported throughout the region. There were hundreds of after-shocks; dozens of people were injured. This may only be the beginning of a series of potent Southern California earthquakes.

Clark and Carver claim that the potent quakes occurring in the Cascadia zone will be entirely different than the ones which usually afflict the West coast. Most quakes arise from an epicenter, radiating laterally to affect specific regions. The quake predicted by Clark and Carver is called, technically, a subduction zone quake and will potentially affect "tens of thousands of square miles" (CNN World News Report, January 10th, 1992). What's more, it is not just California that would be stricken. The Cascadia zone runs through Oregon and Washington all the way to British Columbia. Carver and Clark note that there is definite evidence that the earth plates in these areas are shifting. The latest California quake (April, 1992) provides further evidence for the subduction zone phenomenon; the trembler rocked buildings from San Diego to San Bernardino, a region some 200 miles north of Los Angeles. The fact that this quake was followed some 72 hours later by an potent earthquake in extreme Northern California gives strong support to Clark and Carver's theory. Therefore, it is crucial that people living within the Cascadia zone prepare for the worst. Make no mistake about it, the L.A. basin and Northern California earthquakes of April, 1992 are connected, that is they are no mere coincidence. People must heed these geological warnings and take the appropriate precautions.

The urgency of this danger is why this book is written. The information contained in it will prove invaluable -- and may well be lifesaving -- if and when a major earthquake strikes. Yet, the utility of the Survivor's Nutritional Pharmacy expands over a greater realm than earthquakes alone. Nuclear and toxic chemical releases are even more likely to afflict Americans in terms of mass injury as are tornadoes, floods and hurricanes. This booklet provides data which is useful in each of these crises.

We cannot ignore the facts. The earth is rumbling. It is hot. Is this due to the Greenhouse effect and the loss of the ozone layer? No one knows for sure, but it is likely that this is partly responsible. In an astonishing revelation researchers reported in August of 1991 that the South Pole is shrinking; some 2% of it has melted away. That is a significant percentage. True, episodic fluctuations in the internal or external temperature of the earth and in volcanic activity do occur. However, much evidence points to the fact that the earth's crust is hotter than ever before and that this effect is largely man-made.

The occurrence of a major earthquake in the United States is ripe. In fact, it is over-ripe. It could happen at any time. Would you be ready if it were to happen tomorrow? Most people are entirely unprepared.

The least that can be done is to prepare for medicinal action. This is so you can help yourself, your family, friends and any stranger in need who might cross your path when no other help will be available. For these reasons, it makes good sense to prepare. This is one area where your actions can be productive, as much misery can be prevented and many lives saved through the correct application of survival medicine.

In a major earthquake it is likely, if not assured, that virtually all forms of medical aid that are normal conveniences of life in America will be cut off. Hospitals will be damaged, destroyed or rendered ineffective. Doctors will be isolated and neutralized. Emergency vehicles, such as ambulances and fire trucks, will be stalled. Medicines, pharmacies and pharmacists will be unavailable.

It is clear that the individual must make his/her own medicinal preparations. The *"Earthquake" Survivor's Nutritional Pharmacy* is the tailor-made package that the American public needs. It is the perfect answer for personal preparation for the lay person and professional alike. Every person living in the earthquake zones would potentially benefit, as would those living in tornado, flood or hurricane regions. The pharmacy kit provides safe, effective remedies for the majority of illnesses and disabilities which are likely to result from such disasters.

Over the last few years the earth has provided numerous warnings that geological doom is imminent. Many authorities believe that the most likely site for this catastrophe is Southern California. Others hold that Northern California is the probable region. Alaska too is highly vulnerable, as is Nevada. The 1992 earthquakes are beginning. Besides several small tremors around the globe, a major disaster in Turkey took some 1,000 lives and left nearly 200,000 people homeless.

Three separate damage-inducing quakes have occurred in California in 1991. There was also a significant quake in the Midwest during that year. Several have occurred in Russia and in regions such as Iran, Iraq, China, India, and Armenia. The Indian and Russian earthquakes killed several hundred people.

Much of San Francisco was severely damaged in 1989, and the City has yet to recover. The downtown section of Santa Cruz was leveled. Anyone who has visited this city knows that huge holes in the ground still remain and that many downtown businesses operate out of tents. Watsonville, a small town near Santa Cruz, was essentially destroyed by the same quake. It has yet to be fully rebuilt. People living in California need no further warning. The signs are there for all to see.

There is no sure-fire way to be completely prepared for the consequences of a major earthquake. You could make all the preparation in the world, bury your food, water and Pharmacy in a "safe" place, and the earthquake could destroy that too. However, this is no cause to give up hope and/or fail to make preparations. Odds are that if you survive the initial quake, any efforts at being readied will pay off. Plus, a prepared person is more at ease. A person who fails to give thought to the possibilities and takes no action feels much less secure. He/she will be disoriented, stressed and overwhelmed by fear.

Everyone living in the region will be afraid in the event of a major quake. However, those who are fully prepared will be several steps ahead and will have a sense of calm that will be unavailable to the ill-prepared.

If a major earthquake strikes a heavily populated region of the United States, such as Southern California, it will be a catastrophe of untold proportions. To add to the tragedy, many individuals will be injured or will lose their lives due to a lack of preparation or as a consequence of illnesses that could have been prevented.

A variety of cures and remedies for use in the aftermath of a natural disaster are found within these pages. Everything is spelled out. Even the precise dosages are given. The primary objective is to help each individual take charge of his/her health. There is another major objective. Think how rewarding it would be to help someone else, whether it be a your own child or a total stranger. In contrast, think of how frustrating it would be if you couldn't help. Today, helping to save a life is what makes a person a hero.

The lay person cannot be taught complex life-saving

procedures, wound care or surgical techniques. This book makes no attempt to do so. Rather, it describes methods which a five-year old could master and apply. Additionally, all the prescribed remedial agents are non-toxic. For obvious reasons the use of drugs is avoided. The exception might be topical antibiotics or non-prescription pain killers such as aspirin.

Thousands of remedies are found in Nature. The focus herein is on those which are useful for conditions likely to result from major natural disasters. Therefore, this information is of value for victims of tornadoes, hurricanes, chemical spills and floods as well as earthquakes.

Study this manual. Keep a copy of it handy at home, at work, in the car and, if living in an earthquake zone, buried safely in the ground. Review this material often. Take a course in first aid. As a result you will achieve the security available only to the learned and the prepared.

Chapter 2 Are You Prepared to Survive?

There will be a major earthquake in California, and it will likely occur before the year 2000. Precisely when and where it will happen and how extensive will be the damage, no one knows for sure. It may strike only a certain region such as a section of Greater Los Angeles, or it may cause damage throughout California. Regardless of the specifics, every individual living in California must assume the quake will occur within his/her locale and that it will have a direct impact upon his/her life. In fact, each person living there must realize that there is significant risk for personal injury and even death.

There are other regions in the United States which are vulnerable to the occurrence of major earthquakes. They include Alaska, Washington State, Oregon, Nevada and Utah. The Midwest, too, is vulnerable, and fault lines in certain states, notably Missouri, Tennessee and Arkansas, have recently become active. Even the Northeastern States are vulnerable. A major earthquake striking that region measuring greater than 6.0 on the Richter Scale is regarded as a "near certainty" by the end of the 20th Century.

This concern about major natural disasters is not a matter of thinking of the worst. It is a matter of preparing for the most difficult, tenuous and threatening of all situations. People must take the necessary steps to protect themselves. If they don't, they put their lives and, ultimately, the lives of others at risk.

It is true that the great quake may not happen in your lifetime. However, what if it does? Will you be prepared? If it were to happen tomorrow -- would you be ready? It happened in San Francisco, and the people there were ill-prepared. Hundreds of individuals were forced to live in poorly equipped shelters for days. In some cases people lived in their own backyards for days or even weeks. To this day many remain homeless in that they have yet to return to their original homesteads. In spite of the fact that these and other hardships resulting from natural disasters are being faced by Americans seemingly on a daily basis, few people in this country consider that this could ever happen to them. The majority of people living in the earthquake zones give little or no thought to preparing for a major earthquake. They let the days pass by without considering that they too could be displaced from their homes by a sudden geological cataclysm. The same is true of the majority of people living in regions frequented by other natural disasters. Few people living in the vicinity of nuclear plants give thought to preparing for the worst nor do those living near chemical factories.

This manual is about survival. It is designed for individuals bent on surviving and helping others survive: thus its subtitle, "The *Survivor's* Nutritional Pharmacy." In the event of a cataclysm of Nature, it is a system for helping people *stay alive* once they make it past the initial disaster.

Simply put, if you survive a major earthquake or any other catastrophe, you're going to need the Survival Medicine Kit described in this booklet. Its components may mean the difference between life and death; between misery/pain and relief/calm. Having cared for yourself, you may then be able to help save the lives of others. However, you can help no one if you are seriously ill or emotionally out of control.

People living in urban America have little or no knowledge of the healing potions of Nature that are useful for survival. The average person would be lost if left to the elements. Most people would have difficulty telling which way the wind is blowing, which way is east or west, what plants are poisonous or which might be edible, and what to do for injuries. Without the conveniences of modern life, the majority of people would be entirely lost, confused, angry and/or frustrated. Unless cared for, many would fail to survive. This is certainly true of the elderly and infirm. Imagine what would happen if they were left to the elements, wandering about for days, suffering from heat exhaustion, exposure to wind, excess sun or cold, thirst and hunger. It is unlikely that they would last long.

Fortunately, in most major disasters, there are ways that stranded, hurt or lost people can be cared for. In America there exist numerous emergency aid groups: the National Guard, the Coast Guard, the police force, the paramedics and the firemen. However, with a disaster of the magnitude predicted for California, there is no guarantee that any such help will be available. Emergency aid personnel may themselves be among the quake's victims. Truly, there will be no one to rely on. Each individual will be on his or her own, and it is best to prepare for this scenario in any case.

An earthquake can destroy an entire city. What kind of National Guard force would be needed to take care of that?

People cannot blindly hope for or rely on others for relief, rescue or cure, whether they be the National Guard, armed forces, paramedics, firemen, doctors or any other group. Every individual must be prepared to fend for himself/herself and to take the appropriate remedial action. People have a responsibility to do so, for proper preparation will save lives.

Let's look at a likely scenario. You are in your home with your daughter. Suddenly, there is a violent jolt; the world seems as if it is coming to an end. The walls begin tumbling down all around you. In a reflex manner, you grab your daughter and run out of the house. As you rush out, the house crumbles; glass shatters and flies all over. Miraculously, you make it outside safely. You slap yourself on the face and hold on even more tightly to your daughter while trying to make sure this isn't some horrible dream. Yet, it is real, and you know it. After the shock leaves, you notice something very frightening: bright red -- it's blood -- and it's all over you. You search yourself for its source; your hands are covered with it. Then you realize it's not from you; it's from your daughter. Blood is gushing from her upper arm, apparently the result of a cut from flying glass. As your daughter, like you, is in shock, she hardly feels it. Then, as she realizes your concern and feels the pain, she begins to cry.

In a major earthquake this scenario will be all too real. What do you do now, call an ambulance? In all likelihood there will be no ambulances. You think of rushing to the phone but realize there is no phone service; the power lines are down. There will be no rescue of any type, no life-saving helicopters, at least not for some time. You look around and scream for help; no one responds. Acting on reflex, you think of jumping into the car and taking your daughter to the hospital. You rush in the direction of the garage, but there is no garage left, and the car is crushed and buried under the rubble. You dash toward the street only to find it filled with more rubble, downed power lines and splintered trees. Finally, you become despondent and realize that now *you* are the survival expert. You rip off a portion of your shirt/blouse and tie it around the wound, hoping to stop the bleeding.

Individuals trained in backyard survival will take a slightly different approach. This scenario of human injury will be shocking to them too but will not come totally as a surprise. They are prepared for it mentally and medicinally. They know precisely what they can and cannot do. They know that if the wound is too deep or if it involves a tear of a major artery, it may be beyond their ability to control. However, since most wounds are superficial, they have prepared for these more likely circumstances.

In the example previously given, even though blood is gushing forth, the major arteries are intact. The survival-minded parent, having rehearsed this scenario, would rush to the backyard and recover the Survival Medicine Kit. He/she would find within it all that is needed to cleanse superficial as well as many deep wounds. The kit even contains a natural substance which may help control the bleeding. There are gauze pads, cotton balls, tape and bandages. A variety of antiseptics useful for preventing wound infection are found therein. Water is buried nearby. The wound is rinsed to remove dirt, dust and germs. Antiseptics are applied, and the wound is carefully dressed. The parent is surprisingly calm through it all, as is the child; for they are informed, readied, knowledgeable and prepared.

What a difference there is between these two examples. The key to this difference is that the people in the latter example are not caught totally by surprise. They are rehearsed for action. Can you imagine what the performance would be of a football team if it failed to prepare? A basketball or baseball team? A debate team? A spelling bee contestant? A medical or legal student taking exams? Anyone involved in critical events becomes nervous, apprehensive and worried if ill-prepared.

Those living in earthquake zones would be well advised to prepare for an earthquake of the magnitude illustrated by the aforementioned example. Every day, thousands of people methodically prepare for important events. What could be more important than preparing for the disaster of the century?

The objective of the survival natural medicine program is not to teach people how to become trauma experts. That is nearly impossible. Trauma experts tell us that lay people, in their zeal to be helpful, often do more harm than good to individuals with serious injuries, particularly those suffering from spinal cord injuries. We need not attempt heroics.

On the other hand, there are thousands of situations when people can be hurt further or become ill if action is not taken. It is true that the loss of limbs, bleeding from major arteries, broken vertebrae or shattered limbs, blunt trauma or similar catastrophic injuries are all likely to occur in the event of a massive earthquake. However, a greater percentage of survivors will suffer from less severe injuries, such as cuts, bruises, contusions, concussions, uncomplicated fractures and abrasions, than from life-threatening trauma. What's more, evidence exists that the greatest health risks develop after the quake. Experts predict that a greater number of fatalities and sicknesses will result as a consequence of post-quake accidents, toxic fume inhalation, consumption of contaminated water and wound infections than from the more sudden injuries occurring during the initial moments of the earthquake.

Thus, making it through the earthquake or, for that matter, any other type of major natural disaster is only a fraction of the problem. Surviving afterward is the real test. Remember, there will be no electricity, running water, freezers, refrigeration, gas, light or heat. Transportation will be halted. Emergency rooms and hospitals will be incapacitated, and doctors and nurses will be unavailable. No ready-care centers will be ready. Chiropractors and pharmacists will be beyond reach. The circumstances will involve little more than the individual against the elements. As the saying goes, "It will be every man for himself."

The Aftermath

One of the most common causes of death after a natural disaster strikes is infection. Exposure to the elements may also cause deaths, but this mainly affects the infirm, the elderly and children. However, infection can kill anyone, even the most vital and healthy of us.

In a major earthquake there may be an additional cause of fatalities: toxic fume, chemical and/or radiation exposure. The likelihood of significant toxic releases is exemplified by the rash of recent "accidental" chemical spills occurring throughout the United States. Still, infection will be high on the list, and, if the disaster is extensive and the lifestyle disablement prolonged, infection is likely to overcome toxic exposure as the number one cause of post-quake fatalities.

Numerous types of infections must be contended with in the aftermath of a major natural disaster. The most obvious is infection in wounds. This will be exceedingly common following a massive earthquake, as many of the injured will be unable to access adequate medical care. The fact is only a minority of people will receive immediate treatment. Plus, as has been mentioned, there may not be any running water to cleanse the wounds.

The communicable infections are another major concern. Particularly worrisome are the so-called water-borne diseases such as dysentery, cholera and hepatitis. All can, through epidemics, wipe out people by the hundreds or even thousands. These diseases commonly occur in the aftermath of natural disasters.

Viral and bacterial infections develop as a consequence of stress and exposure. Stress may precipitate throat infections and/or the common cold. More significant infections include bronchitis, pneumonia, influenza and urinary tract infections. Each of these illnesses can become life-threatening, particularly in the elderly and children.

What can be done to prevent these infections? First, we must prepare for the worst. We take a crash course -- the thorough reading of this book would serve as one -- on natural medication for survival. In addition, proper wound care and first aid must be learned. However, it is not enough to simply read this book and/or other relevant materials. You must act upon the information.

Remember, the responsibility for survival falls on your shoulders alone. No one else will bear this burden, not the government, municipality, police force, firemen, army, not even your spouse. The individual alone must take the necessary precautions for post-quake survival. He/she must make provisions for the battle ahead, a war fought in a different kind of jungle: the backyard.

Chapter 3 Natural Remedies for Treating Infection

When considering the concept of a medicine kit for treating infections, the first thought that usually comes to mind is the use of the standard antibiotics and antiseptics that can be found in any pharmacy. Unfortunately, antibiotics are only a small part of the answer, and drug store antiseptics are almost useless. Antibiotics are drugs and are available by prescription only. Doctors know the indications for their administration: the public doesn't. It is realized that many people do self-medicate with antibiotics. However, in a disaster situation this will probably cause more harm than good. The antibiotics will likely be ineffective against the specific infectious agents and, in some instances, may actually encourage their growth.

Bacterial infections are the only type which respond to treatment with antibiotics. These drugs do nothing to combat infections by viruses, fungi and parasites.

When an individual is infected in a survival circumstance it is virtually impossible to determine exactly what the causative organism(s) is/are. Medicating oneself with antibiotics is like trying to kill an elephant with a bow and arrow. Thus, a self-limiting infection can be turned into a raging, life-threatening one by the indiscriminate usage of prescription antibiotics.

Antibiotics are a poor choice for topical use on wounds, scrapes or cuts. When an open wound is contaminated, any number of organisms can infect the tissues. This contamination is especially likely if the wounds are touched by human hands, particularly someone else's hands.

The most effective anti-infective agents are those which kill a large variety of organisms. That is why the use of prescription antibiotics is not recommended. They kill only bacteria and then merely certain types. Plus, bacteria can develop resistance to these agents, and they can also develop resistance to most of the standard germicides and antiseptics. A safer and more versatile treatment is the use of various natural compounds known to kill almost any type of microbe, while blocking the development of resistance.

Saving the Best for First: Pure, Raw Honey

One of the most powerful antiseptics known to mankind is not produced in chemistry labs. It is a substance made by bees: pure, raw, honey. Bees are among Nature's finest chemists. Their most abundant production is honey, that sweet substance of varying taste, color, and aroma. They also synthesize bees' wax, royal jelly and propolis.

To many people it may seem astonishing that something so sweet could also be such a potent antiseptic. After all, honey is a food, not a drug. Let's review the relevant history and chemistry in attempt to understand how this could be true.

Bees are gregarious creatures. They live as a colony in close proximity to one another. Anyone who has seen a picture of the inside of a hive knows how tightly packed bees are. Can you imagine what would happen if infection developed within the hive? Once a single bee is infected, the whole clan would rapidly become decimated. Not surprisingly, bee hives are normally sterile.

What keeps the hives sterile? First, the bees' foods are sterile: bee pollen, royal jelly and honey. When bees make honey, they secrete within it natural antibiotic-like substances, increasing its anti-microbial action. Plus, they fan the moisture out of the honey in order to eliminate any possibility of it holding infection. What happens is that the elimination of moisture from the honey causes a change in its chemistry.

This is through the phenomenon of *osmosis*. Osmosis represents a process by which water or other fluids either move toward or away from an area. Honey, being free of moisture, draws water to it. Looking at this another way, if you were to take a tub of water and place a semi-permeable membrane across it, you could create an experiment in osmosis. If salt were added to one side, that would make the water highly osmotic. In other words, water from the unsalted side would be drawn across the membrane. That is why people who are stranded on the oceans die if they drink salt water; it will suck what little water they have left in their bodies right out of them.

The same chemical tendency is true of honey. It craves water by a powerful osmotic effect. However, unlike sea water, it is non-toxic.

Microbes are nearly 90% water, and this is precisely why honey is so antagonistic to them. It literally drains the water and, therefore, life right out of them. Honey is exceptionally effective against bacteria and parasites, since they are mostly water. Plus, raw honey contains natural antibiotics which help kill microbes directly. Yet another important function is that honey, when applied topically, speeds the healing of tissues damaged by infection and/or trauma. It contains vitamins, minerals and enzymes, as well as sugars, all of which aid in the healing of wounds.

The osmotic powers of a substance are directly related to the size and total amount of molecules it contains. Distilled water, which is free of all particles, has no osmotic pull. In the case of plain salt water, it is the sodium and chloride that are responsible for the osmotic effect. With sea water, sodium, chloride, sulfur, manganese, silicon, potassium, magnesium, zinc, copper, cobalt, nickel, boron, vanadium, aluminum, silver, gold and dozens of other molecules are involved. Sea water is one of the most powerful osmotic agents known. Yet, honey is an even more potent osmotic agent. With honey, it is sugar molecules that generate the osmotic pull. These sugars are far larger molecularly than the minerals, and this fact accounts for their exceptionally potent osmotic capacities.

Honey has been used in medicine for centuries. Russian surgeons, prior to the advent of antibiotics, applied raw honey to wounds after surgery, finding that infection was curbed and the rate of healing increased. They used honey to draw pus out of wounds and applied it to infected tissues, such as boils and cysts, successfully destroying these infections. Currently, British doctors are using honey on open surgical wounds, as they too have found that it prevents infection and speeds the healing of wounds. Unfortunately, the vast majority of medical professionals have no knowledge of honey's astounding medicinal capacities.

After reading these fascinating documents, I experimented with raw honey on myself and also on patients who had localized infections. The illnesses treated included boils, acne, cysts, dog bites, cuts, bed sores, burns and abrasions. In every case, the application of raw honey produced positive results. Often, infection was eliminated literally overnight. The honey applications caused the infections to come to a head, drawing out pus and secretions as well as accelerating wound healing.

Decades ago American surgeons have found honey to be of value. They used it post-operatively to pack wounds, noting that localized post-operative infections were essentially eliminated. Plus, wounds healed more quickly with less scarring. Few if any American surgeons currently utilize it. This is unfortunate, since the application of honey on wounds would serve to reduce pain and suffering as well as save limbs and lives.

The primitives have utilized honey as a medicine for centuries. Honey was discovered in the tombs of the pharaohs, and, although it was nearly 4000 years old, it was still edible. The ancients used it as a digestive aid, and there is evidence that they applied it topically to wounds. The physicians of ancient Greece prescribed it often and used it as a carrier for many of their medicines.

The prophet Muhammad (7th century A.D.) was the first to note the tremendous value of honey for the treatment of diarrhea. It is reported that he was extremely fond of honey and often ate it by the pound. Even the most stubborn cases of diarrhea responded to his prescription. More recently, the *Journal of Pediatrics* found honey considerably more effective than glucose syrup in the treatment of diarrheal illness in infants.

All of the holy books speak of honey in "glowing" terms. The Bible glorifies it frequently, mentioning it as a food of the prophets and the heavens. The Qur'an praises it as "a medicine for all mankind."

Truly, for the disaster victim, honey is a cure-all. It is easy to preserve and store, requiring no refrigeration. It will hold up to extremes of heat and cold while still retaining its nutritional value and antiseptic qualities. A tightly sealed jar of honey is one medicine the elements cannot destroy.

What is Pure, Raw Honey?

The kind of honey that is used makes a difference in terms of achieving optimal curative effects. Like any other food, honey can be processed. That processing may destroy its active ingredients. The key is to find honey which undergoes minimal heating, therefore, the designation of *raw*. A second designation is *unfiltered*. Bee keepers often heat and filter honey to make it more "appealing" to the consumer. Heating prevents honey from crystallizing and increases the ease at which it can be removed from the hives. Filtering removes particulate matter that might cause the consumer to be concerned about "purity." After all, who would buy honey in the supermarket that was filled with tiny yellow, brown and/or black particles?

Crystal-clear, highly purified honey is not the type needed for survival. Only unheated and unfiltered honey can be relied upon to get the job done.

The primary reason commercial producers heat the honey to high temperatures is to sterilize or "pasteurize" it. This is unnecessary, as there are no microbes in honey. The only way microbes can get into it is from contamination by human hands after it is extracted. Even then, these microbes will immediately be destroyed by the raw honey's osmotic powers.

The pasteurizing temperatures often exceed 180 degrees Fahrenheit. Honey which is heated gently, up to 130 degrees, still retains most if not all of its biological activity. Heating the honey to high temperatures causes the destruction of vital elements which are responsible for its capacity to heal wounds, kill infections and soothe internal organs. These elements include vitamins, minerals, enzymes, antibiotics, bioflavonoids and organic acids.

Filtering eliminates another vital component: the pollen. Pollen acts as a digestive aid and is a source of quality nutrition, primarily in the form of B-vitamins, protein and nucleic acids. In a crisis situation people will need as much nutrition as they can get. Additionally, the protein in pollen stimulates wound healing when applied topically and also when taken internally.

Honey as a Food

Honey is unique as an earthquake survival aid for several reasons. First, it is a food which cannot spoil. Because of its high sugar content and the powerful osmosis this creates, no microbes can live in it. As long as it is sealed, it will last through floods, quakes, storms or any other natural disasters and still retain its potency. Secondly, it can be eaten by newborns, infants, toddlers, teens and adults alike. The only exception would be diabetics.

Honey's versatility as a food is largely a consequence of the fact that it is predigested. All of the sugars, pollens, enzymes, vitamins and minerals in honey have been acted upon by digestive enzymes from bee saliva. The value of this is that almost no energy from our bodies is required to digest it. Many people notice that they become fatigued after eating. This is due in part to the fact that up to 50% of the energy produced by the body is consumed by the digestive processes. In contrast, the consumption of honey will likely give us a boost in energy. We need to conserve our energies in times of crisis. Honey is the safest and most nutritious blood sugar fix and is an effective body energizer. It is certainly superior to candy as a source of sugar.

Honey consists primarily of sugars, which make up some 80% of its weight. Vitamins and minerals are found only in trace amounts, the exception being darker honeys, which are rich in potassium and other minerals. However, its content of anti-microbial compounds is significant. Honey contains a number of potent bactericides. Even though they occur in only trace amounts, they are highly active against a variety of microbes, including staph, strep and Candida. This may be one reason honey has been used as a vaginal implant, i.e. despite its high sugar content, it inhibits the growth of yeasts. Other studies have shown that it is active against a variety of intestinal pathogens, including Salmonella and Shigella, both of which cause potentially life-threatening diarrheal disease.

Additionally, honey contains a number of organic acids, and these also inhibit bacterial growth. Organic acids are potent germicides which are active against microbes, even in trace amounts. This type of potency for antimicrobial agents should not come as a surprise. Household germicides are often so potent that only a few drops in a bucket of water are sufficient to kill germs.

Enzymes are another component found in trace amounts.

These highly active molecules serve several valuable functions, including aiding in the destruction of microbes, acceleration of wound healing and the facilitation of digestion. Dozens of enzymes are found in honey. Many are so unique that their structure and biochemistry remain unknown.

Honey as an Internal Medicine

Honey is a time-proven remedy for treating diarrheal diseases of all types. Its greatest benefits are seen in infants and children, although it is also effective for adults and the elderly. It usually takes longer for results to be achieved in older people, with the most rapid responses seen in infants. The elderly simply respond and heal more slowly due to sluggish immune, hormonal and digestive functions.

Medical professionals might wonder at the audacity of recommending an innocuous food substance like honey for the treatment of potentially serious conditions. Many would resist the idea that honey is a cure for diarrhea, and others would deny it outright. Yet, what cures has the medical profession offered for diarrhea? Lomotil (Imodium)? Kaopectate? Pepto Bismol? Antibiotics? Clear fluids and bed rest? None of these come anywhere near matching the effectiveness of honey.

With diarrhea honey cures through a mechanism that is logical. Honey is so readily digested that its sugars are immediately absorbed into the bloodstream. Once there, the sugars act to increase the osmotic pull of the blood, preventing water from being lost into the small intestine and colon. In diarrhea it is not the intestines that are losing the water; it is being lost from the tissues and blood. Remember, honey is water-attracting. It helps the tissues retain the water in addition to another group of critical components: the electrolytes.

Electrolytes are a special category of minerals which are

crucial for survival. They include sodium, potassium, iodine, chloride, magnesium and bicarbonate, a non-mineral substance.

Whenever fluid is lost from the body, electrolytes are carried with it. That is because water is a solvent. Pure or distilled water is unknown to our bodies. The water within us, which constitutes some 70 percent of our total weight, consists of a mixture of compounds, including electrolytes, major minerals (zinc, copper and calcium) and vitamins. When water is lost, so are all of these components.

Millions of people throughout the world die from diarrheal diseases every year. Several thousand of these deaths occur in the United States. Here, Salmonella infection, food poisoning and intestinal flu are the main causes. In the rest of the world, Shigella infection, intestinal worms, amebic dysentery and cholera are the primary causes. Many people die from the loss of electrolytes, which causes hypotension (low blood pressure), cardiac arrhythmia and sudden death. Others die from malnutrition and dehydration.

It is crucial to stop the diarrhea before fluid and electrolyte losses become extreme. Diarrhea constitutes a net loss of fluids and electrolytes from the bloodstream and tissues, into the intestines, and out of the body. That is the definition of dehydration in terms of diarrheal disease. This loss of fluids and electrolytes is the cause of death from diseases of poor sanitation such as dysentery and cholera.

When consumed, honey acts as a suction, causing the blood to retain fluids and electrolytes. Additionally, it acts directly on the intestinal walls to stabilize them against fluid loss. Honey is far superior to the standard remedies for diarrhea such as Pepto Bismol and Kaopectate. The active ingredient in the latter is clay. Comb honey is one of the most effective types, because it is the purest form available. You can't be fooled with comb honey in terms of heating and processing. Heating melts the comb, so if the comb is intact, the honey is 100% pure. Even so, many brands of quality raw honeys with the comb removed are available.

I have utilized honey with great success for the treatment of diarrhea secondary to intestinal flu and food poisoning. Thus far, every case has responded positively. This may seem astonishing, but, knowing the physiology of diarrhea, it makes sense that honey will ultimately cure the condition. The raw honey treatment works even in the most stubborn cases. If it appears that the individual is failing to respond, the amount of honey consumed should be increased. It is often necessary to consume as much as a pound of honey per day in order to stop the diarrhea. This amount of honey is harmless, except in diabetics. The diarrhea is what will kill us. People think nothing of consuming a pound of chocolates in a day or for several days in a row in an addictive craze. Some people eat a half pound or more of white sugar every day usually as hidden sugar in their foods. Eating honey in large amounts should not be a concern.

How to Use Honey

For external use the protocol is simple: generously apply the raw honey to the wound with a butter knife or applicator. Continue this treatment two to four times daily. Pack the honey firmly into or against the wound by pressing with gauze pads. Then cover the region with gauze and tape securely.

For internal usage the amount consumed depends upon the individual's age and the severity of the illness. The effectiveness of honey in diarrhea is greatly enhanced if the stricken individual fasts of all solid foods. This allows the honey to work directly upon the area of damage: the gut wall. If possible, one should eat nothing but honey and, for fluids, sip on juices, broth and water. This approach should be followed for the first 12 to 24 hours at a minimum. It may be necessary to continue this broth, juice and soup diet for as long as 72 hours, and solid foods should be limited to fruits and possibly cooked cereals. Additionally, any solid food which is eaten must be chewed well.

The honey should be consumed in amounts as large as is necessary to cause a reduction in the diarrhea. Improvement is measured by a decrease in the frequency of stools, the amount of fluid/stool lost and the degree of intestinal cramping.

The minimal dosage for adults is 2 tablespoons six times daily, although as much as 1/4 cup four to six times daily may be needed. The rule is that more is usually better, since diarrheal diseases threaten lives, and the objective is to stop the loss of fluids and electrolytes as quickly as possible. For children or infants, a tablespoon 4 to 6 times daily should suffice. It is advisable to continue consuming honey even after the diarrhea has stopped in order to prevent a relapse. An excellent maintenance dose would be two tablespoons each morning.

Honey may also prove effective for another serious condition: congestive heart failure. This life-threatening illness occurs primarily in the elderly. It can often be kept under control by medicines but may be precipitated by stress. Can you think of a greater stress than a massive earthquake, where all you have ever built or owned is destroyed? In the congestive heart failure victim, unless he/she is diabetic, raw honey in the dose of 1/4 cup three to four times daily may act as a lifesaver when no doctor can be found.

Burns may also respond positively to the application of honey. This is due to the nature of honey's osmotic effect. When applied to the skin it prevents the loss of tissue fluids, which is a major problem in burn injuries. Additionally, it helps prevent the microbial overgrowth that inevitably occurs in severe burns. Honey is also an excellent remedy for sore throats. It soothes the throat in the case of infection or toxic chemical/smoke inhalation.

Antibiotic Honey From New Zealand

The country of New Zealand is, in fact, a huge island located to the east of Australia. From this repository of Nature comes Manuka honey, one of the most powerful antiseptic honeys in the world. Manuka honey exhibits unusually strong antimicrobial activity. What is most astounding is that it maintains this effect even after being heated. Manuka honey is so potent that it kills staphylococcus, one of the most difficult, hardy bacteria known. Researchers have identified a variety of active ingredients, including powerful aromatic acids, which are found in this type of honey in high amounts. These acids create a low pH which prevents bacterial replication. Manuka honey also contains a considerable amount of hydrogen peroxide. This potent antiseptic kills microbes on contact. Manuka honey is available from Comvita and may be purchased in fine health food stores and specialty shops.

Mountain Honey from America's Deserts

Another exceptional type of honey, Questa honey, is made closer to home in New Mexico. Here, some 8,000 feet above sea level in the high desert mountains, the bees gather the nectar from flowers and clovers which are free from pesticides, herbicides and other chemical contaminants. Thus, Questa honey comes from one of America's purest wildernesses.

Questa honey is unique in that it is guaranteed raw. This means it undergoes no processing that might damage the various healing agents within it. The texture of this honey makes it easy to apply to the wounded area. Its delightful flavor makes it a pleasure to eat, and even those who avoid consuming honey fall in love with it. Both Manuka and Questa honey may be ordered by calling (800)-243-5242.

How to Store the Honey

People living in earthquake zones should bury a large plastic or metal container of honey in their backyards. Additionally, it is advisable to keep a tightly sealed container of honey in the car. If the honey crystallizes, don't be concerned; it is still effective. To liquefy, simply place it in a pan of hot water for several hours or set it out in the sun.

Bee Propolis: Antibiotic and Anti-inflammatory Agent

Bee propolis has been used in the treatment of disease since ancient Grecian times. Many people are aware of how other bee products, such as honey and pollen, are produced. However, few of us comprehend the origins of bee propolis. Bees are primarily gatherers but are also synthetic geniuses. They make honey from the nectar they gather from the fruits and flowers of plants. Bees also collect and process propolis.

Propolis is defined in Webster's dictionary as "bee glue." It is actually a resin, a sticky substance found within the buds and bark of trees and shrubs. Bees gather it for use as a cement in their hives; in a sense, they do use it as a glue. Poplar trees serve as the primary source of propolis.

Propolis serves several crucial functions. It strengthens the structural components of the hive so it can withstand the forces of nature: wind, rain, sleet, snow, hail, heat, cold and storms. By acting as a sealant, it helps prevent other insects from invading the hive and contaminating it. Additionally, it inhibits microbial decay. This is one reason hives stay intact for many years after the bees abandon them.

Bees use propolis to coat any foreign objects which enter their hives, including the bodies of insects or small animals. Astonishingly, a mouse was once found in a bee hive. After stinging it to death, the bees coated the mouse with propolis, a process which kept it virtually intact from decomposition.

As a result of its preservative action, propolis helps keep the hive sterile and, therefore, safe as a haven for the bee colony. Remember, as many as 50,000 bees may live together in a single hive, shoulder to shoulder. The spread of infection would swiftly destroy the colony.

Propolis is a potent natural antibiotic, and its effects are broad-spectrum. It can kill all types of bacteria, a characteristic which makes it superior to the antibiotics of modern medicine. What makes propolis entirely unique is that it is also active against viruses, yeasts, fungi and parasites. Yet, it has none of the side effects of medications, and microbes are unable to develop resistance to it. It is safe to use in large amounts both internally and externally.

Propolis can be used in emergency situations to help coat wounds and prevent infections. In this regard it is ideal for use on minor cuts, abrasions and burns. When applied to these wounds it will reduce inflammation as well as diminish pain.

Localized infections, if allowed to fester, may ultimately result in systemic infections. A systemic infection is defined as a condition wherein bacteria or other organisms invade the blood and/or internal organs. This serious illness is often called "blood poisoning" by the public and is known by doctors as *sepsis*. Without proper medical care, sepsis can prove fatal. The signs and symptoms include fever, sweats, chills, aching joints, headache, rapid heart beat and streaks of redness radiating from the wound toward the heart. If this condition develops and antibiotics are available, it would be wise to take them. However, natural antibiotic agents, such as propolis, should be utilized and can be applied topically and/or taken internally.

Propolis is a phenomenal sterilizing agent. The discovery that bees are relatively immune to infection was first based upon the observation that they failed to decompose after dying. Later, researchers found that bee hives were remarkably free of microbes and that both honey and the larvae of bees were always sterile. Somehow bees become impregnated with substances, propolis being one of them, which repel bacterial and fungal growth. In fact, bee propolis is such a strong preservative that pieces of meat can be preserved from decay when embedded within it.

Alas, our foods are filled with synthetic preservatives, many of which are toxic even in trace amounts, while Nature long ago provided us with safe and effective preservatives of her own. One day it will probably be said, "If we only would have known." However, by then it might be too late.

Survival Usages

Propolis is one of the most versatile naturally-occurring medicinal substances known. The following is a list of the primary usages for propolis in the survival setting:

1. Trauma: Propolis tincture can be sprayed directly on various wounds including burns, cuts and abrasions. In addition to being an antiseptic, it exhibits a mild anesthetic action. This is why it is useful for virtually any type of injury. For children it is ideal, since it doesn't sting.

2. Sore Throat: This is one of the most crucial survival uses for propolis. Spray the propolis tincture on the back of the throat and throughout the oral cavity several times per day. To achieve the greatest results, apply it as soon as the sensation of sore throat begins.

Imagine trying to deal with the added stress of a child or several children coming down with colds, sore throats and/or attacks of tonsillitis. If this happens, therapy should be initiated immediately, before such attacks turn into a full-blown illness. Propolis spray is a prime weapon for preventing sore throats from developing or worsening. Plus, it can be utilized for eradicating infections quickly and completely once they occur. Research and clinical experience have proven that episodes of sore throat and tonsillitis, normally lasting for days or even weeks, can be cured within 24 to 48 hours through the application of propolis tincture. It kills the organisms on contact and also stimulates the immune system to clear the infectious agents from the tissues. Plus, it helps reduce the pain and inflammation, and that can prove invaluable when dealing with screaming, crying, irritable children in a crisis or in any other situation.

3. Wound Healing: Propolis stimulates the regeneration of tissues. As a result wounds heal more quickly and are less likely to become infected. Propolis is one of the richest known sources of *bioflavonoids*, which are among Nature's most powerful anti-inflammatory agents. This is one reason propolis offers unusually potent activity for wound healing and curbing pain.

4. Ear Infections: The application of bee propolis aids in the treatment of infections of the inner and outer ear, as it inhibits the growth of microbes within the ear canal. Apply gauze pads soaked with propolis to the affected region twice per day. Also, spray the back of the throat with propolis tincture, since many ear infections begin there.

5. Corns, Calluses and Other Foot Sores: Bee propolis has been used successfully to treat lesions of the feet. It helps soften corns/calluses and soothes the pain of blisters. This is of major importance for the earthquake situation when the most reliable form of transportation will be a person's own two feet.

6. Toxic Chemicals: Propolis has been found to neutralize much of the toxicity of nuclear and x-irradiation and could be taken internally and applied topically if such exposure occurs.

7. Urinary Tract Infections: Chewing propolis granules or taking propolis capsules several times daily may prove helpful in driving kidney and bladder infections out of the system.

8. Pneumonia and Influenza: Propolis is a potent immune stimulant. It increases the ability of white blood cells to destroy microbes. This function makes it invaluable for the treatment of pneumonia and influenza in the survival setting. These diseases have high mortality rates. Every weapon possible must be used against them. Large doses are usually necessary; take three capsules four times daily, or, if using the tincture, one teaspoon three times daily should be sufficient.

9. Stomach and Intestinal Ulcers: A number of scientific studies have documented the beneficial effects of propolis in the healing of internal ulcers. One study found that tincture of propolis led to an improvement in 90% of the subjects. In several patients, the ulcers healed entirely. Stress plays a significant role in the formation of intestinal/stomach ulcers. A major natural disaster will be an inordinately stressful time, and people with ulcer disease may suffer a relapse. Additionally, new ulcers are likely to develop. The consumption of propolis helps prevent stress-induced ulcers.

Propolis can be found in various forms including creams, salves, lozenges, capsules, pills, granules and tinctures. The Survival Medicine Kit includes propolis as a tincture in a special pump spray bottle. Propolis capsules and ointments are also available.

Tea Tree Oil

Tea tree oil is yet another invaluable antiseptic for the survival pharmacy. This unique substance is created by distillation of the leaves of the Australian Tea tree. Like propolis it is a broad-spectrum antiseptic. Thus, it kills bacteria, viruses, fungi and parasites. However, it is particularly active against fungal organisms of all types, including yeasts.

With tea tree oil a small amount goes a long way, and that makes it ideal for survival. The oil can be applied directly to a variety of wounds and can be used safely within even the deepest of wounds. This usage is particularly valuable when confronted with contaminated wounds which cannot be readily cleansed, such as puncture injuries, especially when medical facilities cannot easily be accessed. One of the major concerns in this scenario is tetanus infection. In the survival setting tetanus shots will be unavailable. If puncture wounds and other deep wounds are saturated with tea tree oil, odds are that tetanus will not develop.

Like propolis, tea tree oil produces a numbing action on wounds. It can be used on wounds in children without causing stinging or irritation. This is true of even the most vicious injuries.

Tea tree oil is a superior antiseptic for use on wounds contaminated by dirt and other debris. In this regard it surpasses all other antiseptics. It penetrates deep into the wound and coats the debris, preventing it from acting as a seed for the maintenance and spread of infection. Of course, every effort should be made to remove as much of the foreign matter as possible. However, this may be difficult to accomplish in the highly unpredictable circumstances of a natural disaster. Additionally, it is important to avoid touching the wound with the hands in order to prevent further contamination.

Tea tree oil has numerous applications in the survival setting. It is highly volatile and, thus, may be inhaled for lung and sinus infections. It can be used as a gargle for throat infections. It is ideal for applying on the gums and teeth in the event of dental infections. For optimal results saturate the involved tooth and the gums surrounding it several times daily.

For women there is a special usage: vaginitis. Nothing

could be more distressing than the added burden of a severe case of vaginal discharge, itching and pain amidst all the other crises. Rub tea tree oil within the vagina two or three times daily. This treatment alone will usually suffice to achieve a cure.

For children with ear infections a single drop can be placed on the outer aspect of the affected ear two or three times daily. Do not drip the oil directly into the ear canal. The vapors from the tea tree oil rapidly penetrate the middle and inner ear, and, thus, its medicinal powers are delivered directly to the site of infection and inflammation. There is an extensive variety of medicinal usages for tea tree oil. It is useful for virtually all types of skin conditions and/or diseases ranging from minor irritations to lacerations, wounds, hives and insect bites. Its indications include cuts, scratches, abrasions, burns, allergic rashes, itchy skin, cold sores, canker sores, psoriasis, eczema, seborrhea, boils, gingivitis, tooth aches, bad breath, toenail fungal infections, fingernail fungal infections, athlete's foot, jock itch, vaginitis, bladder infections, sinus infections, ringworm and acne. Immediate application of the oil effectively neutralizes the toxicity of insect bites, including bee stings and spider bites. It may also prove useful for neutralizing bites by snakes, lizards and other venomous reptiles.

Tea tree oil is Nature's antiseptic par excellence. In the field it is far more versatile than antibiotics. During World War II it was issued in first aid kits to Army and Navy units stationed in the tropics and was found to be so effective that demand quickly outstripped supply. Research has shown that it is such a potent antiseptic that it even outclasses most household disinfectants and germicides in microbial killing power. Some studies have shown tea tree oil is as much as five times more potent than household germicides. It is effective in killing or inhibiting the growth of a wide variety of noxious microbes, including difficult-to-kill organisms such as diphtheria, Aspergillus, Candida, staph, strep, Trichophyton, Epidermophyton and pseudomonas. These actions were studied in the test tube. However, tea tree oil works best on and in human tissues: in blood, pus, dead cells and even dirt.

This substance is ideal for survival. In fact, it is essential to it. You can call tea tree oil the essential oil.

If you are out in the field, be sure to take tea tree oil along with you. You will find it useful for everything from minor irritations or wounds to an itchy scalp, groin and/or vagina. Here is truly a substance that you can't leave home without.

Chapter 4 Injuries

In a survival/disaster setting any type of injury must be regarded as serious until proven otherwise. However, burns are among the most serious of all injuries. They carry the risk of life-threatening consequences: shock and infection. The dangers are greatest for the very young, particularly infants, since even a seemingly small burn affects a proportionally larger surface area. The elderly are also at risk and may rapidly deteriorate when burned.

In the United States thousands of fatalities result from burns every year. Many others die from smoke inhalation. The survivors represent an even greater number: those who are maimed and disfigured by burn-related injuries. This is a problem of considerable magnitude. A natural catastrophe could turn this problem into a monstrous dilemma. The 1991 Oakland fire is one example of the overwhelming nature of massive fire-induced disasters. While modern medicine provides the finest care for the acute consequences of significant body burns, that being the prevention of shock and infection, it offers little for the enhancement of wound healing and prevention of scarring. That is where the remedies of Nature play their greatest role.

There are many variables to consider in natural disasters in regard to the types of burn injuries which may occur. The occurrence of chemical, fire-related, steam, sun or wind burns are all possible. Excessive exposure to sunlight is a major concern. If peoples' homes are destroyed and they don't even have so much as tents to cover them, it wouldn't take long to get cooked by the sun. If all that people have for shelter are the clothes on their backs, getting burned becomes an inevitable circumstance no matter what the color of the skin.

Many states, such as Texas, Arizona and California, are essentially deserts. The sun is powerful, and most people are not accustomed to prolonged exposure. In particular, the elderly and/or children are highly vulnerable for rapidly succumbing to the negative effects of prolonged exposure to sunlight. Heat stroke and exhaustion are possible. The former is often fatal.

What about infants or, for that matter, newborns? Their skin is ultra-sensitive to sunlight. In a short period of time their entire bodies could become sunburned. Full body burns cause great stress within the tissues. Even small burns depress immunity and predispose to infection. Add dry air, dust and inadequate hygiene, and it is easy to see how burns occurring in a survival setting represent a dangerous situation which could lead to health catastrophes.

That is why the Nutritional Survival Pharmacy contains several anti-burn remedies. The most crucial of these is aloe vera.

1. Aloe: This popular remedy is probably best-known as a natural cure for burns and is particularly effective for sunburn. It soothes, heals and cures even the worst cases of sunburn.

A complete nutritional pharmacy would ideally include three methods of aloe application: aloe gels, creams and/or aloe liquid pump spray. The pump spray is excellent for applying a light aloe mist, and the gel and cream are the ideal mediums to use on burns. In the case of sun exposure, the aloe gel can be applied to the skin preventively.

The finest, most effective aloe products are made from the whole leaf. This is because the leaf consists of three parts, all of which contain crucial elements crucial for stimulating the healing process. These parts are the outer rind, the sap and the inner gel. Each of these contain a wide spectrum of compounds which have been proven to enhance the regeneration of damaged skin. The greatest benefit is derived from aloe extracts containing all of these compounds, since they work synergistically.

People are most familiar with the inner gel, since this is the component commonly used in salves, creams and cosmetics. However, the effectiveness of the gel is far less than that of the sap and outer leaf.

The rind and sap contain the vast majority of the anti-inflammatory and antiseptic compounds, for instance, *Lupeol*, which is a pain reliever. *Acemannan* is another valuable component found solely in the sap and rind. According to recent scientific research, acemannan possesses significant anti-viral and tissue healing powers. Hundreds of additional compounds are concentrated in the aloe rind and sap. These include:

trace minerals
mucopolysaccharides
essential fatty acids
vitamins
enzymes
carbohydrates
antioxidants

Only a few companies have produced whole leaf aloe products. Such products are a major improvement over the gel-only approach. Evidence for this is the fact that they may be helpful in the amelioration of a wide variety of illnesses, including burns, digestive disorders, psoriasis, eczema, seborrhea, chronic fatigue and arthritis. Over the past 20 years hundreds of research studies have been performed demonstrating that whole leaf aloe possesses potent anti-bacterial, anti-pain and wound regenerating powers.

Scientists have determined that certain aloe products are as much as ten times more potent in biological activity as other brands. The method of processing appears to be the most crucial factor in preserving the potency of the delicate aloe plant. Thus, while the fresh plant is the ideal source, this is hardly the most practical one for use in a crisis situation.

Over the last 20 years scientists have developed methods for preserving the curative powers of aloe in the forms of aloe gels, creams, ointments and juices. These patented methods involve the extraction of the vital components from the entire plant, a process which captures all of the valuable nutrients found within the central portion of the leaf, or jelly, and those found within the leaf itself. In fact, these scientists have determined that the greatest percentage of healing components is found just beneath the skin of the plant and that the center or jelly portion is the weakest part.

There is a wide variation in the range of prices for aloe products. The higher quality products tend to cost more, since they use larger amounts of aloe leaves per bottle. In comparison, inexpensive products contain only small amounts of the active ingredients of the aloe leaves. The increased potency seen with high-grade aloe products more than compensates for any higher cost. The result is that burns and other wounds heal more rapidly. Plus, scarring is greatly reduced.

32-X Aloe Cream is one example of a quality whole leaf aloe extract. It is the most concentrated product for topical use currently available and is, therefore, ideal for use in the Nutritional Pharmacy. Liquid aloe concentrates for internal use (*Aloe Ace; Coat's Aloe*) are also available (see Appendix C).

In the survival setting, burns may occur as a result of fires as well as accidents such as the spilling of hot water. Chemical burns are also likely to occur in the aftermath of an earthquake. Noxious chemicals can burn the skin either by direct contact as liquids or via exposure to their gaseous forms. The gases pose the greatest danger, as they may burn the internal tissues such as the lungs and mucous membranes as well as the skin.

Billions of gallons of gaseous chemicals are transported in the U.S.A. by rail, pipeline or tanker truck every week. These chemicals include chlorine dioxide, bromine gas, arsene gas, sulfur dioxide, hydrogen sulfide, liquid nitrogen, liquid oxygen, liquid hydrogen, hydrochloric acid, nitric acid, anhydrous ammonia and hydrogen cyanide. All of these compounds rapidly form gases when exposed to air and many are highly flammable.

Violent natural disasters greatly multiply the potential for major toxic gas releases, which are occurring on a monthly basis throughout this country without any provocation from Nature. As scary as it is, at least one minor or major toxic gas release occurs in this country every day.

All of these various types of burns are treatable with aloe jelly, cream or liquid. For internal burns drink the aloe juice. For external burns, apply the aloe to the involved site several times each day and also at night before sleeping. Aloe helps prevent the burns from becoming infected and will minimize, if not eliminate, scarring. For additional scar-blocking effects, liberally apply vitamin E to burned skin.

Radiation poisoning can also cause burns or, more commonly, a type of skin inflammation known as x-ray or radiation dermatitis. Numerous studies indicate that crude aloe extract is a highly effective treatment for this condition. As demonstrated by Dr. Thomas Rowe, Professor of Pharmacology at the University of Virginia Medical School in his research paper, *Further Observations On the Use of Aloe Vera Leaf in the Treatment of Third Degree X-Ray Reactions*, only the crude aloe extracts containing the healing components of the leaf as well as the inner jelly produced consistent results. Usually, even in the most severe radiation burns, the application of quality aloe products to the injured tissue results in an observable difference within hours. Radiation burns can occur in the mouth or other mucous membranes. Aloe is equally effective as a treatment for these lesions.

The aloe extract included in the Survivor's Pharmacy meets the specifications outlined by Rowe. In event of a known radiation release, aloe can be applied in a preemptive attempt to protect the skin from radiation toxicity. Aloe is non-toxic, so it can be applied repeatedly to the skin without concern.

2. Organic Sulfur: Sulfur is another valuable anti-burn remedy. In the Nutritional Pharmacy, sulfur is provided in a unique form: sulfur drops. This type of organic sulfur contains a wide variety of biologically active sulfur compounds. It does contain traces of naturally-occurring sulfites, so it must not be used by asthmatics or other sulfite-sensitive individuals. Simply apply several drops of sulfur to the affected region(s). Or, add it to the aloe gel and rub the mixture on burns and into wounds. Sulfur helps reduce swelling and pain in injured tissues, as it is one of the most potent natural anti-inflammatory agents known.

The aloe/sulfur mixture makes an excellent burn ointment. It may also be used for the topical treatment of severe allergic rashes such as hives and poison ivy.

Many people are likely to associate organic sulfur with the drug of similar name, *Sulfa*. While hundreds of thousands of Americans are allergic to Sulfa drugs, allergy to organic sulfur is rare, the exception being those who are highly reactive to sulfites.

3. Tea Tree Oil: Besides shock, the major concern of trauma experts in regard to major body burns is infection. Infection is the major cause of fatality in those who survive the initial stages of burn injuries. Once infection occurs in patients with major body burns, it is extremely difficult to control and/or eradicate. These patients are at high risk for the development of a variety of systemic infections as a consequence of shock,

impaired circulation, tissue destruction and immune depression.

The skin is a most crucial defense for preventing the human body from invasion by noxious microbes. It is a formidable mechanical barrier. Additionally, the skin contains a variety of substances which inhibit the growth of microbes. These include fatty acids and naturally-occurring flora. Additionally, the layers just under the skin provide immune surveillance. If microbes begin to invade the skin, chemicals within it send messages which provoke an immune response. Usually, the invading organisms are destroyed by the white blood cells which, through their ameba-like action, are capable of squeezing into the skin layers. Or, the infection is "walled off", and, thus, systemic infection is prevented.

Body burns, even relatively minor ones, alter immune function. The more significant burns cause a profound depression of immunity. After massive body burns occur the tissues remain sterile for, at the most, approximately 24 hours. However, this is merely the calm before the storm. Massive microbial growth begins to occur. This makes sense. There is no longer a mechanical barrier; the skin is destroyed. So too are the locally-occurring white blood cells. The central immune function is severely depressed, and the adrenal glands are failing. The circulation is impaired and the nutrient reserves of the tissues have been exhausted. A most frightening circumstance has developed: there is dead skin everywhere, a perfect medium for the growth of microbes.

In the event of a major natural disaster it is reasonable to presume that such body burns may occur when no medical expertise can be procured. No ambulances can be summoned, no Life Flights can deliver and no drugs can be prescribed.

While there is little that lay people can do to treat the shock suffered by burn patients in the field, there is a great deal that can be done to prevent infection. As was previously stated, we have approximately 24 hours to prevent infections from developing. If nothing is done the dead skin will feed whatever microbes it comes in contact with. Soon, microbes infect the damaged outer tissues in staggering numbers, up to several million per square centimeter. If left unchecked they invade the deeper tissues, ultimately gaining access to the blood. This is called sepsis, and in the field it will be uniformly fatal.

Are antibiotics the answer? They may be helpful, but they are not the cure. The problem is that the skin is usually infected by a variety of antibiotic-resistent organisms, including Proteus, Staph and Pseudomonas. Additionally, fungi, notably Candida albicans, readily infect burned tissues, and the consumption of antibiotics only serves to encourage their growth.

Burn victims are in dire need of a topical antiseptic which, while being non-toxic to the traumatized tissues, will prevent infection from developing within these tissues and also effectively treat it once it occurs. Tea tree oil fits this description.

Amazingly, applications of tea tree oil can help keep burns sterile, preventing the damaged tissues from acting as a seed for the growth of microbes. Additionally, as was mentioned previously, research indicates that it increases the rate of healing, aiding in the formation of new skin cells and decreasing scar tissue formation. Apply the tea tree oil as soon as possible after burns occur. As always, avoid direct contact of human hands with the burn sites. Drip the tea tree oil from a sterilized dropper bottle, or apply it to sterile dressings. However, in most instances, burns heal best if they are left undressed.

Eye Injuries

Each of us has only two eyes. In an earthquake there are numerous scenarios for eye injuries: flying glass, foreign objects, dust, chemical burns, ulcerations and dryness due to exposure. Under these pressures and stresses, the outer eye may become damaged to the degree that infections develop. That could spell trouble when living outdoors and fighting the elements.

Just think -- for those who wear contact lenses, how will they be kept sanitized? If a person is outdoors all day with winds blowing and dust flying, the eye membranes will eventually become dry. Plus, it is likely that people will be dehydrated so that there are no tears to keep the eyes clean. Dry eyes plus contact lenses spells trouble. Scratched corneas, irritation and infection are all likely to occur.

Aloe vera is one of the most reliable, versatile remedies for the eyes. As long as it is kept sterile it is safe for use in the eyes. Aloe is an unusually gentle herb. It is the ideal agent for the treatment of chemical burns of the eyes.

Alex Duarte, a California optometrist, has found that aloe is extremely effective for the treatment of damaged and/or irritated eyes. Abrasions of the cornea from contact lenses respond particularly well. Says Dr. Duarte, "The cornea is the fastest healing tissue in the human body... When the cornea is scratched some of the cells will travel like amoeba to the damaged area and fill the abrasion." He has found that aloe vera applied directly to the eyes increases the effectiveness of this natural healing process. He also prescribes aloe vera in drop form for dry eye syndromes. According to his prescription, the drops must be administered several times per day for optimal effects.

Burns of the eyes, whether accidental or due to sun or wind exposure, must be treated to prevent corneal scarring. Aloe vera is perhaps the most reliable treatment in this situation. If the aloe is applied immediately after the injury and regularly thereafter, odds are that scarring will be prevented or minimized, and the vision will remain intact. As always, be sure to flush the eyes thoroughly with water in the event of chemical eye burns. In addition, the aloe will soothe the pain with its cooling and numbing actions.

If the eyes are burned by acids, flush repeatedly with large amounts of water. If little or no water is available use any type of ingestible fluid you can find, including milk and/or juice. Additionally, acid burns may be neutralized by mild bases (i.e. baking soda) and burns by bases with mild acids (i.e. vinegar and/or lemon juice). However, adding such compounds to the eyes is dangerous. That is because the interaction between acids and bases always gives off heat and the added heat may serve to make the injury worse.

Follow all flushings with a solution of aloe extract and water. To reiterate, the flushing solution of choice is pure water, and neutralization should only be attempted if water or other compatible fluids are unavailable.

Vitamin A

Vitamin A is probably the single most important nutrient for the maintenance of healthy eye tissues. It is the key nutrient responsible for night vision. Thus, it would not come as a surprise that night blindness is due primarily to a vitamin A deficiency. Other nutrients required for proper night vision include riboflavin, vitamin C, bioflavonoids, folic acid, magnesium and zinc.

In dropper form Vitamin A can be used to help speed the healing of outer eye injuries. It may also aid in the treatment of eye infections, since vitamin A is one of the eye's natural antibiotics. Our tears contain a certain amount of it.

In the Nutritional Pharmacy vitamin A is found as vitamin A drops. This is a detergent-free water-soluble type of vitamin A, which is ideal for application as drops into the eye. Most water-soluble vitamin A products contain traces of detergents, which are utilized in the manufacturing process. These detergents irritate the eyes and remove the protective natural compounds which coat it. One drop of detergent-free vitamin A three to four times daily is sufficient for the treatment of most eye conditions. For those suffering with night blindness, five to ten drops may be taken internally for several days or until the night blindness improves. Reduce the dosage to one or two drops daily, as vitamin A does accumulate in the body and an excess can cause toxicity. However, water-soluble vitamin A is the least toxic type.

Vitamin A controls the rate of cellular growth. Whenever tissues are damaged, great stress is placed upon the involved cells and organs as well as upon supportive organs throughout the body. Supportive organs which are involved in the healing process include the pancreas, liver, adrenal glands, thyroid gland and immune system. Stress and injury cause an increased need by cells and organs for nutrients, especially those involved in tissue regeneration. Such nutrients include vitamins A, C, E, B-2 (riboflavin), B-5 (pantothenic acid), B-6 (pyridoxine), folic acid; amino acids and fatty acids; and the minerals copper, manganese, sulfur, silicon and zinc.

These nutrients stimulate wound healing and. They be taken internally or applied topically. Vitamin A drops can be applied to superficial wounds anywhere in the body but should not be utilized for deep wounds. For minor cuts, wounds or abrasions, one or two drops added directly to the injury site each day should be sufficient.

Vitamin A acts, in a sense, as a form of natural cortisone. It reduces inflammation and lessens scar formation. Unlike cortisone, it improves local immunity, decreasing the risk of infection. Cortisone tends to depress immunity and delays wound healing. Vitamin A has no ill effects upon wound healing. Thus, it offers all the positive benefits of cortisone without the drawbacks.

It is easy to comprehend how rapidly the human body can break down in times of trial and stress, such as in the aftermath of a major natural disaster. This is a time when few of the normal conveniences of life are available. People who have experienced such disasters can readily relate to these words. We live in a convenience society and are not accustomed to any disruption in the usual flow of things.

In the aftermath of a major earthquake nutrition may be less than adequate, and the stresses will be greatly heightened. Vitamin A is a crucial anti-stress nutrient and is found in fresh foods such as meats, milk, butter and eggs. It is also found in fresh dark green leafy vegetables and yellow-orange fruit/vegetables as beta carotene. In the event of a major natural disaster it is likely that vitamin A deficiency will develop, since the availability of fresh foods may be entirely curtailed. People will become deficient in a matter of days, except for experienced hunters who are able to kill wild game and eat the internal organs. This is how the primitives got their vitamin A. The internal organs, the greatest natural source of vitamin A, are the first things the mountain lion, bear, wolf or any other carnivore eats when it kills its prey.

Vitamin A deficiency impairs immunity and impedes wound healing. Thus, it greatly increases the risks for the development of serious infections such as diarrheal diseases, pneumonia and influenza. Prolonged stress alone causes Vitamin A deficiency. Add to that poor diet and a super-deficiency state will likely develop. Symptoms of deficiency include:

night blindness
dry scaly skin
brittle fingernails
hair loss
dry or brittle hair
diarrhea
acne

loss of smell
loss of taste
loss of appetite
fatigue
dermatitis
susceptibility to infections
weight loss

Bone Injuries: Fractures, Bruised Bones and Sprains

Can you imagine how common and debilitating bone injuries will be in an earthquake? Every type of injury ranging from sprained ankles to torn cartilage and complicated fractures will occur. Nothing in this manual can prepare the general public for dealing with life-threatening medical emergencies such as would be seen with severe fractures. However, people can be prepared to deal with less severe injuries such as sprains, minor fractures (without dislocation) and bruised bones.

There are three key approaches to such injuries: *rest, reduction* of inflammation and *rebuilding* of bone and other damaged connective tissues (i.e. ligaments, tendons, etc.). Remember this as the R.R.R. rule.

Rest is simple enough. Reducing inflammation involves a two-fold approach: that which can be applied topically at the injury site and that which can reduce inflammation through internal consumption.

Bromelain: Nature's Anti-inflammatory Agent

Scientific studies have shown that bromelain, a natural substance found in the stems of pineapples, reduces pain and inflammation as effectively as many anti-inflammatory drugs, including aspirin. Bromelain is safer to use than these drugs and can be taken in relatively large amounts without ill effects. Aspirin, which is one of the weakest of the anti-inflammatory drugs, cannot be taken in large doses without the risk of significant side effects. The only exception for bromelain's low toxicity is allergy; people who are allergic to pineapple may also be allergic to bromelain. However, the number of people allergic to aspirin is far greater.

Bromelain reduces the swelling typically occurring in acute injuries, such as an ankle or knee sprain, something that aspirin cannot usually do. The ultimate result is less pain and quicker healing.

Most of the bromelain currently available in the marketplace is enteric coated. This is done on the supposition that bromelain, being an enzyme, will be destroyed by stomach acid. The coating is an attempt to get the bromelain to pass through the stomach intact so it can be absorbed in the small intestine. Unfortunately, this coating is often so firm that the bromelain never completely dissolves and is lost in the stool. Bromelain which is un-coated is absorbed far more easily, and stomach acid apparently does not inactivate it. A typical dosage is two to six tablets taken several times daily (i.e. 500 to 1500 milligrams). Continue this dosage until a noticeable improvement occurs. Then reduce the dosage to a maintenance level of one tablet three times daily.

Technically, bromelain is classified as a proteolytic enzyme. This means that it digests protein. Injured tissue consists of dead and damaged cells, which are mostly protein, and various inflammatory proteins secreted by cells in response to injury. Bromelain helps process these proteins so they are less toxic to the injury site. That is why bromelain may prove helpful for a wide range of traumatic injuries, including fractures, bruises, swellings, sprains, cuts and burns.

All traumatic injuries have one thing in common: swelling of the tissues (edema). This swelling, though a normal, physiological response to trauma, is a nuisance in respect to the healing process. The edema presses on nerve fibers, causing pain and impedes blood flow, which slows the rate of healing. To enhance the rate of healing and diminish pain, it is essential that the swelling be reduced and/or eliminated. Bromelain is perhaps the most versatile natural substance in this regard. Scientific studies document its amazing effectiveness at reducing the edema that results from burns, blunt trauma, fractures and lacerations. In addition, it helps increase blood flow to the traumatized region. The result is a measurable increase in the rate of healing.

There is an additional use for bromelain: blood clots. Bromelain is a natural "Roto-Rooter" agent, functioning to dissolve clots in arteries and veins. Blood clots are a common consequence of massive trauma and are especially likely to develop in the event of complicated fractures and blunt trauma. These clots may travel to the lungs, liver, heart or brain, causing heart attacks, liver infarctions, pulmonary infarctions, pulmonary emboli and/or strokes. Infarction is defined as massive cell death. Thus, blood clots are a major cause of fatalities in trauma patients. Bromelain's value is two-fold: it helps prevent the occurrence of clots and dissolves them once they occur.

In summary, bromelain may be used in the treatment of virtually any type of injury or inflammation. It is a safer, more reliable choice for the treatment of acute injury than aspirin or Tylenol.

Helping to Rebuild Bone: The Calcium Connection

When and if a major earthquake strikes, fractures will occur in great numbers. Some of these will be so severe as to ultimately cause death. Untreated fractures may also lead to the loss of limbs. However, the majority of fractures will be of the non-life-threatening variety albeit, no doubt, painful and debilitating.

When people think of bone, they usually conceive of it as it exists on a skeleton: dead. In reality, bone is living tissue and is constantly undergoing change. It is subjected to stress on a daily basis and is affected by lifestyle habits, including exercise or a lack thereof, alcohol consumption, drug usage, smoking and diet.

Many people have weak bones. However, even the strongest bones cannot withstand the trauma of heavy falling objects, motor vehicle accidents, falls from heights and similar trauma.

If the trauma is severe enough fractures are inevitable. However, if they occur people must do everything conceivable to help their bodies heal the damaged tissue as rapidly as possible. That is where bone-building nutrients come in.

Women are particularly vulnerable to fractures, and this is especially true of elderly and/or post-menopausal women. Hip fracture is one of the most common causes of traumatic injuries in post-menopausal women. This type of fracture, which occurs in hundreds of thousands of elderly women every year, will be exceedingly common in the aftermath of a major earthquake. Even minor falls could cause hip fractures in susceptible individuals.

After bone injury occurs, much can be done to ensure and accelerate healing. Since bone is living tissue it, like all other tissues, is dependent upon sufficient nutrition for adequate growth and repair. The most critical elements for the repairing of bone are protein and minerals, although certain vitamins also play important roles. Thus, as a start, a multiple vitamin/mineral plus extra vitamin C will help accelerate healing. The most important vitamins for bone healing are vitamins A,C,D and K. Vitamin D is involved in calcium absorption and metabolism. Vitamins A and C enhance the formation of bone protein and its cellular cement, the *mucopolysaccharides*. Minerals provide the bedrock for bone support and are crucial for reconstruction. Sufficient protein is also needed. The bones consist largely of protein, and it is protein which gives them their flexibility. Thus, in the event of a fracture, protein intake should be increased.

However, the single most important nutrient for fracture repair is a substance called *microcrystalline hydroxyapatite* (MCHC). In actuality, this is the same material found in our bones and is responsible for the maintenance of bone strength. It consists primarily of calcium and various bone proteins.

MCHC is an effective remedy for the repair of bruised and broken bones as well as sprained joints. Studies have shown that this compound accelerates the healing of damaged bones and joints, including arthritic ones. In some instances new cartilage was formed in the joints as a result. Therefore, it would also be ideal for injuries involving cartilage damage such as sprains and torn ligaments.

MCHC is an extract from the bones of young animals. It is never heated and is in essence a raw compound. That may explain why it is so effective, since it is an entirely natural, unaltered supplement. The typical dosage for sprains and other minor trauma is 6 tablets per day. For broken bones, 12 to 15 tablets may be taken daily. People with large bone mass must take greater amounts than those with small bones. For children, 5 tablets daily is usually sufficient. There is one minor side effect of these large doses; in certain people, constipation may occur.

Calcium is found in the diet in relatively few foods. Milk, cheese, yogurt, canned fish and dark green leafy vegetables are the primary sources. Additionally, carrot juice contains a considerable amount. These foods will be difficult to procure in times of crisis. Hence, the value of maintaining a sufficient stock of calcium supplements and MCHC is emphasized.

Fractures can be best diagnosed by one simple test: the bearing of any amount of weight by the involved bone(s) will be inordinately painful, if not impossible. Again, it is impossible to turn lay people into expert medical diagnosticians. Suffice it to say that if a fracture is suspected and no medical help can be procured, splint the region and immediately begin therapy with MCHC as well as other nutrients. A dosage of 15 tablets daily for the first 72 hours after the injury occurs would be advised.

The final step in joint or bone treatment is topical application of substances which reduce pain, swelling and/or inflammation. One could apply the propolis spray, aloe gel or an herbal liniment to the involved region. The Nutritional Pharmacy prescribes a unique vitamin C cream. Called Derma-C, this cream contains special components which cause the vitamin C to penetrate deep into the traumatized region. This leads to a reduction in inflammation and pain while speeding the rate of healing. Vitamin C may be useful for the variety of minor injuries typically occurring in earthquakes. These include bruises, contusions, abrasions, lumps on the skull or other bony parts and minor cuts. An additional benefit would be protection against skin damage from the sun's ultraviolet rays. Vitamin C has been shown to help skin cells regenerate after exposure to UV light.

For optimal benefits it is important that the vitamin C penetrates into the deepest layers of skin. Studies on Derma-C cream have shown that the vitamin C may be so well absorbed that blood levels may actually be increased after application of this product to the skin.

Major Trauma

Bleeding: Can it Be Stopped?

Unfortunately, there is no 100% foolproof method for stopping bleeding in the field. Success depends largely upon the seriousness of the wounds and whether major arteries have been severed. In addition, the problem of internal bleeding is an extraordinarily serious and very realistic concern. Blunt trauma, the primary cause of internal bleeding, commonly occurs in earthquakes. It is almost impossible for the lay person to determine the scope of such trauma, much less do something about it. Obvious symptoms of internal bleeding include blood issuing from the mouth, vagina, penis or anus and/or a drop in blood pressure or pulse.

The Astounding Miracle of Liquid Trace Minerals

Liquid Trace Minerals are the closest thing to a survival anti-bleeding agent short of a tourniquet. This natural compound is invaluable for use in the field during a major natural disaster. In such circumstances people will need as many miracle workers as possible.

Liquid Trace Minerals is a blackish-brown fluid consisting of a variety of inorganic minerals. It arises directly from the earth, in fact, deep inside it. It is mined from the Florida Everglades where liquefied mineral deposits were produced as a consequence of the decay of living matter over millions of years. The minerals are highly concentrated in this formula, just as they are found in nature. Analysis of this blackish-brown fluid reveals an unusually high content of iron, manganese, silicon, magnesium, copper and untold other minerals.

What is so fantastic about the Trace Mineral solution is that, when applied to superficial wounds, it stops bleeding on contact. Although the mechanisms are unknown, it is likely that this effect is due to a unique combination of minerals or possibly the type of minerals found within it. Regardless of the reason, the Trace Minerals quickly coagulate blood without causing toxicity.

This product is most effective for controlling bleeding

from minor wounds: for example, scrapes, abrasions or superficial cuts on the hands or arms. In more involved wounds, it may impede the rate of bleeding when no medical personnel or facilities are available. It may also help slow or curb internal bleeding.

With superficial cuts or abrasions it is possible to actually see the blood congeal after applying the Trace Minerals. However, it should be reiterated that the first step for treating a seriously bleeding wound in the field is the application of pressure, either on the artery above the wound or directly over the wound with a pressure bandage. There may be need for a loose tourniquet, although most emergency medical authorities warn against its use in the field. After all standard measures have been exhausted, apply the Trace Minerals.

Liquid Trace Minerals cannot stop bleeding from a severed major artery. The only solution to that is surgery. Yet, wounds of a lesser degree occur more commonly, and that is where the Trace Mineral solution finds its optimal use. It is ideal for application to lacerations of the scalp, face, neck, arms, legs, hands and feet. Simply drip the Trace Minerals on the bleeding region repeatedly until the blood firmly coagulates. For stubborn wounds, apply gauze pads soaked with Trace Minerals and tape over the wound. Or, preferably, apply steady pressure with the Trace Mineral-soaked bandages until bleeding stops.

An additional benefit is that the Trace Minerals aid in wound healing. The minerals contained in it form a part of every cell, whether arterial, muscular, venous or skin, and this fact probably accounts for much of its healing potential. This compound also acts as an anti-microbial agent, and its regular use will help prevent wound infection. The Liquid Trace Minerals are one of the most important substances to keep in the vehicular and home nutritional pharmacy kit.

Chapter 5 Internal Disorders

Nausea

To be in pain is miserable, but to suffer with nausea is often even more distressing. This is because nausea represents a combination of a sort of pain plus a sickening, an almost indescribable feeling. Being nauseated truly represents one of life's most uncomfortable sensations, and with all the other stresses to confront in a natural disaster nausea is the last thing anyone will need.

Nausea can often rapidly be cured. The most valuable remedy for treating it is a common herb and: ginger. This root, which is used as a spice in everything from bakery to stir fry, has an astounding ability to curb nausea. While its mechanism of action has yet to be determined, research indicates that it reduces inflammation in the stomach wall and also within the liver. Since nausea is often related to liver function, it is likely that ginger exerts its action by stimulating and/or enhancing the liver's functional activities. This may also be why it is so highly regarded for use in cooking; it serves as a digestive stimulant. Regardless of the mechanism, an emergency pharmacy cannot be without it. The simplest way to store ginger is in the form of capsules of the pulverized dried root.

In most instances three capsules taken several times per day will help to curb the nausea. Larger amounts can safely be consumed if necessary. For children open the ginger capsules and stir the powder in water or juice. Make it into a tea. This remedy works well for most types of stomach pain or nausea, but, again, repeated use may be necessary.

Acidophilus supplements may also prove helpful, as nausea can be a consequence of microbial overgrowth in the stomach or intestines. Take 1 or 2 capsules morning and night with meals. Additionally, if the nausea is severe, fasting is indicated. Solid foods should be avoided, while soups, broths, water and juices should be consumed.

It must be emphasized that nausea may be a sign of serious diseases. These diseases/conditions include gastrointestinal bleeding, peptic ulcers, hepatitis, cancer, brain tumors, stroke, heart attacks and head injuries. The use of ginger root is limited to non-pathological conditions such as nausea of pregnancy, stress-induced nausea and that which occurs in people suffering from migraines, diarrheal disease or motion sickness.

Hepatitis

There will be big trouble in the aftermath of an earthquake when the water mains burst. The water from the faucets, if any faucets still work, will become brown. It will look like muddy water. That's what happened in 1989 in San Francisco and Santa Cruz. It is what happened in April, 1992, in Guadalajara after the sewer system exploded. Drinking water will be mixed with dirt and probably raw sewage. Anyone who drinks this water is at risk for developing a very serious and potentially fatal disease: hepatitis.

Hepatitis is defined as inflammation of the liver. That inflammation may be caused by exposure to toxic chemicals, alcohol consumption, drugs or, more commonly, infection.

It has been known for decades that the most common source of infective hepatitis is fecal to oral transmission. The hepatitis virus may live within humans. It may enter the sewage system and be dispersed into the waterways and soils. However, it usually doesn't cause infection unless people are directly contaminated by fecal material or water containing it. Improper hand washing after defecation is known to spread hepatitis, and workers in restaurants can transmit this disease to diners in this manner. Infections may be contracted from the consumption of raw seafood, since the oceans are continually being contaminated by human wastes and shellfish concentrate these. For instance, the cholera/hepatitis epidemic in South America has been traced to the consumption of raw or improperly cooked oysters and clams.

Infectious hepatitis is most commonly caused by viruses, and there are several types. They include hepatitis A, B, non-A/non-B, and the newest type, hepatitis C. These viruses are the most common cause of viral hepatitis, although other viruses such as CMV, Epstein-Barr, rubella, HIV and herpes may infect the liver.

Hepatitis is commonly known *yellow jaundice*. Jaundice is due to the accumulation of a yellowish pigment called *bilirubin*. This is a normal by-product from the breakdown of dead or diseased red blood cells. Normally, bilirubin is detoxified by the liver and will not accumulate within the body in sufficient amounts to turn people yellow. In hepatitis the liver cells are damaged, and, often, a large percentage of the liver mass is destroyed. The result is that the bilirubin processing capacity is disrupted and it no longer can be adequately eliminated.

All of the nutrients described in this book aid in the prevention and treatment of hepatitis. Of exceptional value is a substance called *beet root flavonoid*. Beets help heal the liver, but a person would have to eat a few bushel baskets full to achieve the desired results. Fortunately, the technology exists to concentrate the active principles of beets, and that is precisely what beet root flavonoid is. A teaspoon of this remarkable compound is equivalent to several pounds of beets in terms of therapeutic value. If stricken with hepatitis, take a heaping teaspoonful of beet root flavonoid several times each day along with other liver-healing nutrients, including vitamins A, B-complex, C, and E, glutathione, zinc and selenium. The jaundice should improve within 48 hours.

Liv-52 is another exceptionally valuable substance. It is a combination of herbs found to be effective in the treatment of hepatitis. Studies have shown that this herbal supplement helps prevent liver damage and also increases the capacity of liver cells to regenerate after damage occurs. Other natural compounds which aid liver function include chlorella, dandelion root, ginger root, garlic, onion, aloe vera, silymarin, black radish root, turmeric, biotin, lipoic acid, N-acetyl cysteine, lecithin, choline and methionine. Numerous scientific studies have documented a positive benefit of chlorella in the reversal of chemical-induced hepatitis, and choline, N-acetyl cysteine as well as lipoic acid have also been utilized for this purpose.

Antiparasitic Agents: *The Value of Organic Sulfur*

Today, doctors use sulfur to treat a variety of illnesses, including allergies, hair loss, intestinal parasitism and vaginitis, to name a few. Sulfur has been used as an anti-parasitic agent since ancient times. The Greeks used it for treatment of a variety of parasitic diseases, including dysentery and scabies.

Do you remember the horrible smell of rotten eggs in chemistry lab? That's the smell of sulfur. Just imagine how parasites react in the presence of this horrid smell; it drives them right out of the system. All kidding aside, sulfur is toxic to a variety of parasites, including Giardia, trichomonas, amebas and various intestinal worms.

When sanitation is non-existent, as would be the likely circumstance in the aftermath of a major earthquake, parasites of all types will have a heyday. These include worms, protozoans and amoebas.

Giardiasis is the most commonly occurring protozoal

infection in America today. It is responsible for hundreds of thousands of cases of diarrheal disease every year. However, infections by intestinal worms and amebas represent a significant cause as well.

Sulfur, in the form of organic sulfur drops, may prove invaluable as a general, non-toxic agent for destroying a variety of parasites.

The standard dosage for sulfur drops is 10 to 12 drops in fluid or placed in a gelatin capsule twice daily. In the event of severe parasitic infection with uncontrollable diarrhea, take 18 drops twice daily. This dosage should be continued for three to five days.

Other valuable uses for sulfur relate to its ability to accelerate wound healing. A few drops can be used to coat wounds; apply it once or twice daily. Saturate bandages with liquid sulfur; it will soak into the wounds and help prevent infection. Sulfur is an important component of healthy skin. The skin incorporates the sulfur for use in building new skin cells. Thus, it can be applied to irritated or infected skin lesions and may be used along with aloe vera to help soothe and heal burns. The combination of sulfur plus aloe makes what is probably the most effective burn regenerating ointment known.

Intestinalis: The Antiparasitic Herbal Formula

It is well known that herbs fight parasites. Virtually all of the primitive societies discovered and utilized specific herbs for killing them.

In America today parasitic infection is common. As many as one in five Americans are affected. The parasites belong to a family of rather large and highly invasive organisms called *protozoans*. *Entamoeba histolytica* and *Giardia lambia* are cited as the most common culprits. Eradication of the infections is crucial, since these organisms are a significant cause of chronic ill health. In addition, both Entamoeba and Giardia can cause life-threatening illness. Intestinalis is active against both of these protozoans.

Intestinalis is a combination of twenty-two herbs possessing antiparasitic actions. This formula was developed by Louis Parrish, M.D., who used it in his parasitiolgy practice for many years before making it available to the public. The product is a must for the Nutritional Pharmacy. An appropriate dosage is 2 to 3 capsules three times daily.

Acidophilus: The Helpful Bacteria

Acidophilus can help save lives. Recent research has shown that this bacteria prevents death and debilitation from diseases such as dysentery, Salmonella infection and cholera. Some of this research was carried out in Bangladesh, where thousands die every year from diarrheal diseases.

The helpful bacteria are probably best known as the organisms responsible for the fermentation of milk to yogurt. The health benefits of yogurt are often attributed to its high content of beneficial bacteria.

While it isn't feasible to store yogurt for survival purposes, storing acidophilus is. Today the technology is available for keeping billions of these organisms alive in gelatin capsules, tablets or in powder form.

Why are these bacteria so important? They are one of the most effective defenses against many of the life-threatening infections typically occurring in survival circumstances. These infections may be caused by a variety of organisms, including viruses, bacteria, fungi and parasites. The specific organisms include flu viruses, herpes, CMV, Camphylobacter, staph, strep, E. Coli, Salmonella, Shigella, encephalitis viruses, amebas, protozoans, intestinal worms and yeasts. Infectious diseases, such as influenza, pneumonia, encephalitis, meningitis, blood poisoning and dysentery, all can kill.

Ultimately, all are preventable.

Serious, life-threatening infections are known medically as *systemic infections*. These infections usually begin as localized infections in regions such as the sinuses, intestines, lungs or skin. Under normal circumstances the body's innate mechanisms of resistance keep the infections at bay until the immune system can eradicate them. However, if the immune system is compromised and/or if individuals are under excessive stress, the infection can spread into the blood and internal organs.

Acidophilus, as well as its sister bacterium, *bifidus*, reduces the risks for systemic infections by preventing infections from gaining a foothold. These bacteria are normal inhabitants of the human intestines, skin, vaginal tract and urinary tract. Known as the "good" or "friendly" bacteria, they function to prevent the overgrowth of organisms which have the potential to cause disease. These latter organisms, called pathogens, often live in a repressed state within the human intestine although, in the case of disease, they may be found on the skin as well as within the vagina, kidneys, bladder, lungs, prostate, spleen and liver.

Under normal circumstances, the good bacteria keep these noxious bacteria repressed. One means by which they accomplish this is via the secretion of a variety of antibiotic-like substances which inhibit the growth of pathogens.

The same is true with pathogens that can be contracted from the environment, such as Salmonella and hepatitis, since the real cure is stopping the infections before they become established. Imagine this scenario. The earthquake strikes and water mains are busted. A person unknowingly drinks water contaminated by sewage. The water is laced with a variety of noxious pathogens, including E. Coli, Salmonella, Camphylobacter, hepatitis viruses, amebas, intestinal worms and possibly even the cholera organism. Once this death soup has been swallowed, acidophilus culture may be one of the few effective supplements useful for combating this problem. If a billion harmful bacteria are swallowed, they must be combated by swallowing several billion good bacteria.

The consumption of acidophilus is a realistic treatment. It has been used in dysentery-plagued Bangladesh with success. Studies have shown that diarrheal diseases, such as dysentery and cholera, can be relieved and/or prevented by the timely consumption of acidophilus supplements. In one study, travelers from the Western world were pre-treated with acidophilus for a week prior to taking trips to regions where diarrheal diseases are endemic: Nepal, Guatemala and Mexico. The results of the study showed substantial protection against diarrheal diseases. Only 4% of the acidophilus-consuming participants developed digestive disturbances, while the normal rate of occurrence is nearly 30%.

Without treatment, dysentery may cause death within a few short, miserable hours. Children and the elderly are particularly vulnerable.

Every hour thousands of people die all over the world from diarrheal disease. The saddest part is that many of these deaths could have been prevented.

The experts predict that in the event of a major earthquake diarrheal diseases could claim as many if not more lives than the earthquake itself. One of the most effective preventive measures would be to take acidophilus on a regular basis in order to impregnate the gut with these organisms. In the event of water contamination or sudden diarrheal illness, acidophilus supplements should be consumed immediately in large doses. As many as three capsules every hour may be required in the initial stages. Continue to take the acidophilus in large doses until the diarrhea dissipates, and then reduce the dosage.

Intestinal infection represents a war, the battle being fought between the noxious organisms and the friendly ones. At times it is necessary to provide the friendly bacteria with assistance.

The natural antibiotics prescribed in this book may prove helpful in winning the war, since they kill the harmful bacteria while leaving the acidophilus organisms intact.

However, don't rush to the prescription antibiotics if diarrhea develops. In fact, that would be the worst thing to do. This is because antibiotics destroy both good and bad bacteria. When the good bacteria are eliminated, noxious organisms are more readily able to fill the void and, thus, create an even a stronger base. Instead, take large doses of acidophilus and utilize the other prescribed anti-diarrheal remedies.

Remember, antibiotics kill only bacteria. If the infection is due to parasites or fungi, antibiotics may well turn a bad situation into a total nightmare. This is because antibiotics destroy the naturally occurring inhibitory organisms, particularly acidophilus and bifidus.

The most beneficial acidophilus products are those which contain organisms derived from a special strain known as DDS. This strain of acidophilus has been studied extensively by scientists. It has been found that DDS acidophilus is more likely to implant or inhabit the intestines than those derived from other sources.

The success of intestinal warfare is dependent upon which organism has the greatest capacity to gain a foothold. In other words, which one will gain property rights? Bacteria, as well as most other microbes, achieve this via the phenomenon of *implantation*. Without the capacity to implant, to adhere firmly to the gut wall, bacteria would simply fall off and be passed through our bodies via our wastes. They infect and live only by locking onto our tissues. In some cases they actually invade the cells and live within them.

The war is ultimately won by the organism or group of organisms which most effectively adheres to the tissues. That is how cholera occurs. The comma-shaped bacterial organism which causes this disease possesses an unusual tenacity for adhering tightly to the intestinal walls. Cholera is manifested by severe intestinal cramping, fever, chills and watery diarrhea. Unrelenting diarrhea results in the loss of large amounts of fluids and electrolytes. Death usually results from dehydration and/or cardiac arrest. Cholera can develop only if the organisms are able to bind to the gut in large numbers. That binding will occur much more readily in the unhealthy colon, especially when there is a reduced count of acidophilus bacteria. In epidemics the mortality rate for cholera often exceeds 50 percent. This makes it the most dangerous of all diarrheal diseases.

Prevention is the most valuable usage for acidophilus. This means that it should be taken on a regular basis before a crisis strikes. With DDS acidophilus products, the typical dose would be one capsule taken twice daily.

Acidophilus products are effective only if the bacteria are viable (alive). These sensitive bacteria are rapidly destroyed by heat. Thus, it is necessary to refrigerate acidophilus and store it in a cool place when travelling. Or, as an alternative, stabilized acidophilus products may be purchased. The stabilization process keeps the organisms alive when kept at room temperature. A number of companies distribute "room temperature" acidophilus. In any case, for survival purposes, acidophilus may be buried in a sealed container in the ground, and that will sufficiently preserve the organisms.

Acidophilus bacteria are rapidly destroyed when exposed to air; oxygen is just as toxic to these organisms as is heat. Some firms package their acidophilus in nitrogen-flushed glass bottles. The nitrogen drives all other gases out of the bottles, and, thus, optimal viability of the bacteria is maintained. Vacuum packing also helps ensure viability.

Lateroflora: The Bacteria-Killing Bacteria

No discussion about beneficial bacteria would be complete without mentioning Lateroflora. This bacteria is highly antagonistic to noxious microbes. Researchers have found that it actually kills Salmonella and E.Coli. It is also highly antagonistic to yeasts and parasites.

By clearing out the noxious organisms, Lateroflora serves an immense function: it helps make room for the good bacteria, the acidophilus, making it easier for these organisms to implant. Thus, an ideal regimen would be to consume Lateroflora for several days prior to consuming the acidophilus.

Chapter 5 Antioxidants

Recently, a report was presented in Los Angeles regarding the number of deaths and injuries likely to occur as a result of a massive Californian earthquake. It is estimated that as many as 14,000 people will be killed outright and that 12,000 to 55,000 will be injured seriously enough to require hospitalization. Studies have shown that additional casualties are likely to result from exploding toxic substances, ruptured pipelines, burning tanker trucks/railroad cars and similar sources of toxic compounds.

These predictions are conservative. Some experts have estimated the death toll to be as high as 100,000 and the injured to number in the hundreds of thousands.

What is more important than any numerical prediction is the statement that more people are likely to be killed and injured in the aftermath due to the liberation of toxic fumes, liquid chemicals, radioactive compounds and other industrial poisons than those killed and injured directly by the quake itself. The point is, many of these deaths probably can be prevented and the injuries minimized. Antioxidants are one of the key players in this prevention.

Antioxidants are a group of compounds which function to block oxidative reactions. Thousands of antioxidants are found in Nature. Hundreds of others are produced synthetically. To understand the value of antioxidants, it is helpful to review basic chemistry. Antioxidants work by inactivating or minimizing oxidative reactions. These reactions occur within our bodies by the millions every fraction of every second. Just what are oxidative reactions? Oxidation is a chemical process wherein oxygen interacts with various substances, be they chemical or living, causing them to decay. Thus, the process of oxidation results in the decay of complex substances into simpler molecules.

Imagine what the world would be like without oxidation. Every plant, animal and pile of garbage that ever existed would be heaped upon each other. Nothing would decay. There would be nowhere to live and no room to breathe. Oxidation is, therefore, a necessary and natural process. When a nail rusts, it oxidizes. When our bodies age, they undergo oxidation. When a plants decay, they are being oxidized. However, too much oxidation is harmful, and, in many instances, the occurrence of excessive oxidative reactions causes tissue damage and even death.

What makes the antioxidants so important to humans is that they halt the development of excessive oxidative reactions. They prevent the internal damage that is likely to result from inhaling or ingesting toxic compounds. To a degree they may even minimize the toxicity of radiation, including nuclear radiation.

Is it possible that large segments of the population could become poisoned by radiation. What if nuclear reactors, such as those located along the West Coast, are damaged? What about petrochemical plants? Natural gas explosions? Burning gasoline or oil? Kerosene? Other hydrocarbons? What about the release of toxic gases from damaged chemical plants? Chlorine and bromine gases? Acid gases? Insecticides and herbicides? Anhydrous ammonia? Cyanide, as in Bhopal? Are Americans prepared? Not in the least.

Then there is the possibility of exploding tanker cars, as might occur on the highways and railways. Toxic gases of all types will be liberated: nitrogen dioxide, sulfur dioxide, hydrogen sulfide, ammonia, ozone, pure oxygen, pesticide plumes, bromine and chlorine clouds. These noxious gases can destroy lung tissue within seconds, in fact, within fractions of seconds. People are not prepared for protecting themselves against toxic calamities and are entirely unaware of what to do in the event of such exposures. The people in Dunsmuir, California, were not prepared for metam-sodium. Dozens of local residents filled the emergency rooms, suffering from illnesses due to inhalation of pesticide fumes. No prescriptions or antidotes were available. Instead, the medical profession set up "assurance centers." The Indians slaughtered at Bhopal were ill-prepared, as were the untold thousands who were irradiated by the Chernobyl plant. In contrast, those who study this manual will be prepared, at least for their own protection. A massive earthquake in an industrialized, chemically-infested region of this country has never occurred. In such an instance, anything is possible -- pesticide/herbicide spills, massive toxic clouds, acid spills or clouds of acid gases, petrochemical spills/fires and nuclear releases. No amount of "assurance" will help people feel secure in these circumstances.

Antioxidants to the Rescue

Antioxidants are a class of chemicals which inactivate other chemicals, specifically toxic ones. They are crucial for stimulating the healing of tissues damaged by toxicity and oxidation. Even if people live through the quake and the after-shocks, there is no guarantee that they will be able to out-pace a toxic cloud; and human beings will find nowhere to hide if nuclear radiation leakage occurs.

People throughout the United States who have suffered from the ill effects of toxic chemical spills, those living near Three Mile Island, and, on a larger scale, the victims of the Chernobyl and Bhopal disasters know how true these words are. It would be wise to learn from their tragedies. What is the lesson? Take the necessary steps to ensure that if an environmental catastrophe occurs in your neighborhood you are prepared.

Antioxidants will help give you the best chance of survival. So will a mask.

Most people recall the vivid scenes of a relatively recent example of the havoc wreaked upon the human body by toxic fumes: the Bhopal massacre. This was a major environmental disaster of the 1980's and was the consequence of an accidental release of cyanide in the form of methyl isocyanate, one of the most toxic gases known. It killed its victims through respiratory failure. Simply put, the gas oxidized lung tissue, literally killing the entire lung. Thousands died, most within minutes. The deaths were a consequence of a gruesome and painful suffocation. Uncountable others suffered permanent, debilitating respiratory damage. It is a horrible way to live, having to catch your breath after exertions as minimal as walking across the room. Yet, that is the plight of many of the survivors.

Just think of what could happen if an earthquake ripped through a chemical plant here in the U.S.A. Thousands of people could be acutely exposed to gases which would tear their lungs apart. The toxic clouds could wipe out entire neighborhoods, if not cities. Death would be a consequence of chemically-induced lung tissue damage through the process of tremendous *oxidative chemical reactions*. This is why antioxidants are so important, since they block these reactions, and it is crucial to keep them at ready access. Thus, individuals might also choose to have a kit readily available at work, especially if they live downwind of chemical or nuclear plants, so that all bases will be covered.

What is the first step if an airborne exposure is imminent? Get as far away from the region as you can. Immediately don a mask; a dust or surgical mask would offer minimal protection. If using a surgical mask, use two or even three. If none of these are available, cover the mouth and nose with a handkerchief or towel, or, rip off a piece of clothing. Grab a pair of goggles or glasses. At all costs cover your mouth and nose, because the most potentially damaging route of entry is through the lungs.

Optimal protection would be achieved by purchasing an anti-toxin mask. These highly specialized masks are used in industry to prevent the inhalation of toxic fumes. People living or working near (or down wind of) chemical plants, nuclear reactors and/or railroad tracks should keep one handy at home and in the car. If a toxic release occurs, cover up as much as possible. Put on a hat. Shield your eyes. Stay indoors, or, if possible, leave the area.

Next, grab your antioxidants. Wait a minute. You don't even know what they are and how much to take. To find out, read on.

What Are Antioxidants?

There are thousands of antioxidants. Many are naturally-occurring. Others are synthetic. This book focuses on the more commonly available naturally-occurring antioxidants which are, incidentally, those with the lowest toxicity.

Antioxidants act as shields for cells, protecting them from damage caused by a variety of noxious agents, including toxic gases, carcinogens, x-rays, ultraviolet radiation, petroleum products and nuclear radiation. In particular, antioxidants protect us from reactions within our bodies which generate a highly reactive group of chemicals called *free radicals*. Free radicals are potent, unstable molecules which can damage our cells. As discussed previously, they are produced as a consequence of chemical processes occurring within the body called oxidative reactions. Toxic chemicals produce much of their damage through generating free radicals and by initiating oxidative reactions. In other words, they oxidize human tissue. For instance, if a person gets a whiff of exhaust fumes, ozone, sulfur dioxide or chlorine gas, lung tissue is oxidized and free radicals are generated within the lungs. Radioactive chemicals also oxidize tissues. Ultraviolet radiation from the sun may oxidize the skin.

Stresses of all types contribute to oxidative damage. Examples of these stresses include exercise, emotional stress, pollution, the ingestion of toxic or rancid fats, impaired nutrition and exposure to oxidative chemicals.

Research on Antioxidants

There are thousands of research articles delineating the role played by antioxidants in the protection of human tissues. Researchers have found that much of the toxicity of air pollutants, radioactive chemicals and other chemical contaminants can be blocked by antioxidants. Additionally, if tissue damage does occur, antioxidants greatly accelerate the healing process. Naturally-occurring antioxidants include vitamins A, C and E, thiamine, pantothenic acid, PABA, lipoic acid, riboflavin, beta carotene, selenium, zinc, folic acid, vitamin B-12, cysteine, methionine, coenzyme Q-10, superoxide dismutase, catalase and glutathione. For earthquake survival, vitamin C, vitamin E, beta carotene, folic acid, selenium, zinc and glutathione are antioxidants that people cannot afford to be without. A survival kit including these should be kept at ready access in both the home an in the vehicle.

Vitamin E

Vitamin E is a crucial antioxidant which functions as an internal preservative. Thus, it helps keep tissues "young" from the inside out. Vitamin E exerts this effect by preventing oxidation of the cell membranes. Since oxidation causes aging, vitamin E prevents aging of the tissues.

For survival purposes vitamin E serves several crucial functions. It helps prevent blood clots, which are a likely consequence of severe trauma. Blood clots are a common complication of injuries such as untreated fractures and blunt trauma (crush injuries). In addition, Vitamin E improves blood flow and accelerates wound healing.

However, vitamin E's primary survival value results from its role as an antioxidant, particularly in respect to the lungs. Researchers have found that this antioxidant largely reverses the lung damage that results from the inhalation of toxic gases. As a preventive agent, it strengthens lung tissue and improves the ability of lung cells to survive toxic insults.

Decades ago, researchers found that toxic chemicals, once inhaled, can cause permanent lung damage. That damage includes cell death and the resultant scarring of the lungs. Vitamin E helps prevent lung cell death and minimizes scar tissue formation once damage has occurred. If cell death and scar tissue formation can be minimized or reversed, the lungs can heal to a normal or near-normal state. The regular consumption of vitamin E is an integral part of the insurance plan for the prevention of permanent lung damage.

Vitamin E is also a potent anti-radiation substance. It intercepts radioactive molecules, neutralizing them before they do damage. The greater the radiation exposure is, the more massive is the amount of vitamin E that will be required. If a significant radioactive exposure develops, vitamin E will be used up quickly, since, once it intercepts radioactive molecules, it is destroyed. Thus, in the event of a massive toxic insult, it must be consumed repeatedly day and night. As much as 10,000 I.U. can be safely consumed over short periods as would be necessary to detoxify the initial onslaught of radioactivity. In the event of massive radioactivity exposure, the dosage is 1,200 I.U. every three hours for adults, 800 I.U. for children and 400 I.U. for infants.

Researchers have found that exposure to a variety of

toxins depletes vitamin E levels within the blood and other tissues. The human body is constantly being exposed to these toxins. Thus, vitamin E must be continually replenished. The only way to do so under survival circumstances is via nutritional supplements. Vitamin E cannot be produced by the human body.

What is the ideal daily dose? That depends upon the circumstances and also the individual. For children 400 I.U. is usually sufficient. For adults a minimum dosage of 1200 I.U. daily is advised. However, during massive toxic exposure, particularly nuclear toxicity, consumption of much higher dosages is necessary.

Vitamin E is also an excellent treatment for lesions of the skin. It is an anti-rash, anti-irritation, anti-abrasion, anti-ulceration and anti-burn agent. Rub vitamin E on any type of burn, including sunburn. Apply it a minimum of twice daily. Keep several capsules of all-natural vitamin E in the vehicle and safely stored in the survival kit. To comprehend the definition of all-natural vitamin E, see Dr. Igram's first book, *Eat Right To Live Long*, which is available in many bookstores or, by mail order: (800) 243-5242.

Beta Carotene

Most people have heard the slogan that carrot juice is good for you. It is, but mainly because it contains beta carotene. This is the substance responsible for its orange color.

Beta carotene is probably best known for its role in cancer prevention. What is less commonly understood is that it is one of the most potent of all naturally-occurring antioxidants.

Beta carotene detoxifies the toxic components of oxygen, and oxygen is responsible for much of the damage which occurs in chemically-induced lung damage.

Beta carotene is an anti-radiation substance. In plants it

functions to protect leaves and stems against damage from the sun's powerful ultraviolet rays. It has the same effect in humans, offering significant protection against ionizing radiation from the sun and, therefore, preventing or minimizing sunburn.

Normally, beta carotene is concentrated in significant amounts in the skin as well as in internal organs such as the liver, intestines, adrenal glands, kidneys and lungs. Stress, as well as exposure to sunlight and toxic chemicals, leads to a rapid decline in tissue beta carotene levels. Unfortunately, carrot juice will be an unreliable source in the aftermath of the great quake. You will need to get your beta carotene from condensed, non-perishable sources such as beta carotene capsules.

It is important to increase one's skin and tissue levels of beta carotene for a variety of reasons. This nutrient is crucial for protecting the cell nucleus from being damaged. In other words, it is nature's preservative for our genes. Genetic material is highly vulnerable to damage induced by various types of radiation, especially nuclear. Synthetic chemicals, radioactive materials and toxic oxidative gases, such as nitrous oxide, sulfur dioxide and chlorine dioxide, as well as heavy metals, all induce genetic damage. Much of this damage can be blocked by keeping blood and tissue beta carotene levels elevated and by replenishing it as it is used up.

Beta carotene is relatively innocuous, even if taken in large quantities. However, it is possible to consume too much beta carotene. If the skin turns yellow, it's time to cut back.

Many foods are rich in beta carotene, and these include dark green leafy vegetables, tomatoes, red peppers, pumpkins, yellow squash, carrots, cantaloupe and apricots. Most of these foods would be impractical sources of this nutrient during a major crisis. One food that is rich and which can be readily stored is red hot chili or cayenne pepper. Cayenne pepper is available in capsule form as a nutritional supplement.

Green algae, notably spirulina and chlorella, are excellent sources of natural carotenes and are, pound for pound, among the richest food sources known. Chlorella is the type recommended for the survival kit.

Natural beta carotene supplements, which are more concentrated sources than the algae, are the most practical survival sources for this nutrient. These are made from a different type of aquatic plant, the salt water *Duniella algae*. Most of the beta carotene on the market is synthetic, and this type is weaker in biological effects compared to the natural algal extract. In case of exposure to radiation or toxic fumes take 100,000 I.U. of natural beta carotene daily. For protection from sunlight 50,000 I.U. should be adequate. To achieve optimal protection against a major release of nuclear radiation, 200,000 to 500,000 I.U.'s taken daily would be necessary.

Vitamin C

It has been known for decades that vitamin C helps protect the human body from the ill effects of toxic substances. As an anti-toxin its functions are innumerable. As an antioxidant it helps rejuvenate cells damaged by toxins, drugs, excessive sunlight and microbes. As a chelating agent it binds to toxic compounds, neutralizing them and aiding in their excretion.

One of the most beneficial aspects of vitamin C in regard to survival relates to its role in lung function. It is found in high amounts in lung tissue, as it protects the lungs from ozone and oxygen-induced damage. In fact, vitamin C is so crucial that it is found in lung tissues in concentrations as much as 20 times those measured in the blood.

Vitamin C aids in oxygen transport from the lungs to the bloodstream. In a sense, it helps "control" the highly biologically reactive oxygen molecules, preventing them from inducing cellular injury. It is so important for protecting lung tissue from oxygen and/or chemical-induced toxicity that it is retained by the lungs even when the entire body becomes deficient.

When toxic chemicals enter the lungs, the ability of the human body to neutralize them is directly related to the vitamin C levels within them. The chemicals will cause a certain amount of lung damage, but vitamin C will help minimize it, especially if tissue and blood levels are adequate. However, to keep the damage to an absolute minimum, the vitamin C levels must be continually replenished. The daily consumption of vitamin C supplements would be necessary for this to be achieved.

One of vitamin C's most valuable functions in lung tissue involves its interactions with other antioxidants. It helps conserve, preserve and regenerate vitamin E. In addition, the body's antioxidant enzymes, superoxide dismutase (SOD), catalase and glutathione, are recycled by vitamin C. This illustrates the importance of providing the tissues with as many of the critical antioxidants as possible, since they work together as a team.

Over the last 50 years, researchers have thoroughly documented the tremendous role played by vitamin C in inactivating noxious chemicals. It performs this function through several unique mechanisms. In some instances it deactivates the chemical before it can do damage. An example is the prevention of nitrosamine formation from nitrates. In other instances it aids in the removal of toxic substances from the tissues: for example, the increased excretion of mercury, lead and other heavy metals which occurs during vitamin C therapy. Yet another mechanism is its ability to enhance liver function, a property which indicates that vitamin C aids in the detoxification of virtually all noxious compounds. Lastly, vitamin C protects the cell's metabolic machinery, its membranes and its nuclear materials from the damage which results once toxins enter the body. It also speeds the rate of healing in damaged cells.

Vitamin C exerts significant protective effects on the skin, guarding it from damage due to solar radiation and/or contact with toxic chemicals. Vitamin C cream can serve as a valuable source for the repair of damaged tissue, since it increases both skin and blood levels.

An excellent preventive dose of vitamin C would be 3 grams daily. In the event of toxic exposure, take 8 to 10 grams daily in divided doses. A mild laxative effect is the only likely reaction from consuming such high doses. If this occurs, reduce the dose until bowel function normalizes. Additionally, large doses of vitamin C must be consumed only when fluid intake is adequate, that is 6 to 8 large glasses of water or juice per day.

Fresh fruits and vegetables contain a considerable amount of vitamin C and are the major sources in the American diet. Included are red bell peppers, hot peppers, broccoli, dark green leafy vegetables, Brussels sprouts, red cabbage, limes, lemons, oranges, grapefruits, guavas, strawberries, papayas, melons and currants. Much of the vitamin C content of these foods is lost when they are cooked. For instance, canned spinach contains virtually no vitamin C. Since it is very difficult in a survival setting to get sufficient amounts of fresh foods, it is advisable to take extra insurance by keeping vitamin C supplements safely stored in the car and at home.

Folic Acid

This B-vitamin is of such great importance to human function that an entire book could be written about it, and still the territory would not be fully covered. Folic acid is crucial for the maintenance of healthy human cells. This is largely due to its function in controlling cellular growth. Every part of the cell, the cellular metabolism, the nuclear material, the structure and the immunity, is dependent upon folic acid.

Tissues fail to regenerate unless adequate supplies of folic acid are available. Cells of all types function sub-optimally without it. Damaged tissue is repaired much more quickly if adequate folic acid supplies are available.

In the USA folic acid deficiency is so common that nearly one-half the population has obvious signs and symptoms. These include fatigue, memory impairment, muscle cramps, paranoia, anxiety, headaches, insomnia, hair loss, brittle hair, brittle or slow-growing nails, lack of appetite, headaches, maldigestion, geographic tongue, inflamed tongue and hangnails. Some studies indicate that as many as 90% of Americans consume less than the RDA and are, therefore, folate deficient.

Folic acid is found in only a few food groups, notably muscle meats, organ meats, the germ and bran of whole grains, fresh dark greens, nuts and seeds. Most of these foods will be unavailable during a major environmental crisis.

Studies have shown that large doses of folic acid prevent lung damage due to the inhalation of noxious compounds, including cigarette smoke and air pollutants. Further, these studies have proven that it accelerates lung tissue healing after such damage occurs. Effective dosages are high: 10 to 20 milligrams daily taken in divided doses. Lower doses will also offer protection.

B-12 is the vitamin companion to folic acid and is also needed to optimize cellular growth and wound healing. However, in terms of survival, folic acid is the more crucial of the two. The cells in our bodies tenaciously adhere to vitamin B-12; in addition, the liver maintains a ready reserve. Thus, most people have enough B-12 reserve to last several weeks or months. In contrast, folic acid is rapidly lost from the tissues and must be replaced continually. Plus, it is even more effective in preventing tissue damage and accelerating healing than is B-12. Meats, eggs and milk products are the primary dietary sources of B-12.

Chlorella, a single celled fresh water algae, is one of the few plant sources of vitamin B-12. Folic acid and B-12 are, in essence, a nutritional pair. They work together in assisting the healing process and optimal effects are achieved when they are taken together. Chlorella is the preferred B-12 source, since the vitamin is poorly absorbed from traditional supplements.

Zinc

Zinc is known as the wound healing mineral. Wounds of all types heal more completely and rapidly if adequate zinc is consumed. Whether tissue damage occurs within the body or on the skin, those tissues must be regenerated if normal function is to return. Without zinc, wounds heal slowly and, in some instances, may not heal at all.

Most Americans are deficient in zinc. This is a result of poor dietary habits but is also related to problems with our soils. The topsoil in most states is lacking zinc. Chemical fertilizers tend to bind zinc, making it unavailable to the crops. Soil erosion devastates zinc levels. Thus, the food grown on affected soils is deficient.

Additionally, food processing destroys zinc. Most of the food consumed by Americans is processed. Examples of processed foods include white flour products (white bread, pasta, bagels, buns, pastries, rolls, cereals, pretzels, cookies and crackers), sugary foods (candy, pop, cookies, doughnuts, fruit drinks, popsicles, canned fruits, pies, puddings, cakes, brownies, ice cream), white rice, fast foods and canned foods. All of these foods are depleted of zinc.

Zinc is well tolerated and absorbed when taken as a supplement. The preferable type is chelated zinc. For preventive purposes 30 to 50 milligrams may be taken daily, preferably with meals. Certain circumstances increase the body's demand for zinc. These include stress, drug therapy, malabsorption, infection and injury. If an individual is under stress or suffering with an infection or serious injury, he/she should take 75 to 100 milligrams daily until the condition is resolved. Long-term consumption of large doses of zinc is inadvisable, since excess zinc is toxic.

Zinc plays a significant role in the function of the immune system. In fact, one of the cardinal symptoms of zinc deficiency is heightened susceptibility to infections. Taking supplemental zinc will help keep the immune system strong during times of crisis.

Selenium

This is the most crucial antioxidant mineral for the purposes of survival. Selenium's importance is based upon its function in neutralizing and detoxifying a variety of poisons. It is particularly effective for preventing the toxicity of heavy metals. Additionally, it is highly active against hydrocarbons, including the gases that are released from burning petrochemicals. It is also a potent anti-inflammatory agent and has been found useful in this regard for diseases ranging from allergies to arthritis.

Much of the effectiveness of selenium in neutralizing toxins is due to its role in boosting the synthesis of glutathione, the most abundant antioxidant enzyme in the human body. In fact, selenium is a crucial part of the glutathione molecule, and, without it, this life-saving enzyme is rendered virtually useless.

Selenium is rapidly assimilated, so it will begin inactivating and destroying toxins almost immediately. To keep the lungs, blood, liver, skin, immune system and every other organ system from being damaged irreparably, take selenium at the outset of any toxic exposure and also take it preventively. In the event of a massive toxic exposure, immediately take 1 milligram of selenium, then take 200 micrograms every hour for at least two days. Take 1 to 2 milligrams per day thereafter until the exposure is eliminated or symptoms disappear. Selenium should be consumed during an exposure even if no symptoms exist, because the ill effects may not always be manifested right away.

Hydrocarbons of all types, whether from cigarette smoke, smog or toxic fumes, cause a reduction in tissue levels of selenium. The greater the hydrocarbon exposure is, the more profound will be the selenium depletion. In essence, selenium is used up, or sacrificed, in order to protect our tissues from these toxins. Additionally, this mineral helps reduce the severity of allergic reactions. It can be utilized in the treatment of a variety of allergic reactions and allergy-induced illnesses but is particularly valuable for alleviating chemical and/or food sensitivity.

The Nutritional Pharmacy contains a unique form of selenium for ready use and easy assimilation. The selenium is dispensed in a small dropper bottle which can be stored conveniently in a purse or in the glove box or ashtray of a vehicle. These drops may be swallowed or held for a few minutes under the tongue for direct absorption into the bloodstream. There is a word of caution: it is possible to get too much selenium. However, the recommended dosages are safe if used for the purposes described.

Concerns for the toxicity of selenium are generally overblown and cannot be compared to the life-threatening toxicity of noxious chemicals. In other words, don't worry about taking extra doses of selenium over the short term for fighting chemical exposure.

The type of selenium with the lowest toxicity is organically bound selenium. Chemically, it is the most stable type. In fact, this selenium is essentially non-toxic. Organic selenium products for long-term usage include selenium-kelp and selenomethionine. These forms are found in capsules or tablets and may be more convenient for regular usage than the liquid. These are the preferred types for daily consumption. Avoid sodium selenite. It is toxic even in small doses.

Glutathione

If a single substance had to be chosen for ameliorating toxic chemical exposure, it would be glutathione. This substance is invaluable for the prevention and treatment of illness due to toxic exposures, and this includes any type of toxicity. A variety of substances ranging from drugs and cigarette smoke to pesticides can be detoxified by it.

Glutathione is different from the previously mentioned antioxidants. Rather than being a vitamin or mineral, it is an enzyme. It is one of Nature's most potent antioxidants.

Glutathione serves as the front-line defense for human cells. It helps the cells detoxify all manner of noxious compounds, including radioactive chemicals, toxic gases, ultraviolet light, hydrocarbons, pesticides, herbicides and heavy metals. A partial list of the specific chemicals it deactivates includes:

* hydrogen peroxide
* benzene
* malathion
* lead
* cadmium
* mercury
* arsenic
* chlorine gas
* sulfur dioxide
* sulfites

* hydrogen sulfide
* gasoline (and its fumes)
* cigarette smoke
* alcohol
* x-irradiation
* radioactive compounds
* ultraviolet radiation
* aflatoxin
* aliphatic hydrocarbons
* pesticides
* herbicides
* poisonous plants

Concentrations of glutathione are particularly high in the lungs and liver, and these organs are constantly being exposed to toxic compounds. Chronic or massive toxic exposure leads to a decline in tissue levels of glutathione. Levels may be increased by taking additional antioxidants such as vitamin C, vitamin E or selenium. The latter forms an integral component of the specialized glutathione molecule known as glutathione peroxidase. Selenium is required for the synthesis of this enzyme.

Glutathione protects our cells from all types of cellular injury due to toxicity. It helps prevent human cells from becoming oxidized. We cannot live without it.

Glutathione is a large molecule. Therefore, its absorption may be impaired as a result of intestinal disorders such as colitis, Crohn's disease, diarrhea, ulcers or malabsorption. Only a small amount of an oral dose will be absorbed, and that may be as little as 10%. Even so, that amount is usually significant enough to produce measurable benefits.

Since glutathione is such a crucial front line defense, it is one of the first things to grab if a toxic exposure occurs. Begin with a loading dose of 8 capsules (50 milligrams each).

Then take 4 capsules every three to four hours for at least 48 hours.

Glutathione is an excellent supplement for the treatment of stress-related illnesses. If an individual is under stress, especially if nutrition is impaired, it is a good idea to take 200 to 400 milligrams of glutathione on a daily basis.

Glutathione can also be taken to prevent stress-induced immune damage and to help block allergic tendencies. In addition, it will effectively neutralize jet lag.

Glutathione capsules should be kept handy at all times. A whiff of diesel fumes or cigarette smoke can make susceptible people sick. Glutathione can come to the rescue.

N-Acetyl Cysteine

Serious injuries and/or deaths resulting from toxic chemical exposure are usually the result of irreparable damage to the lungs, liver and/or kidneys. Medically, this type of injury is known as organ failure. To optimize survival, it is crucial to provide these organs with as much protection as possible.

When the human body is poisoned, regardless of the type of toxin involved, the greatest burden is borne by the liver. This is because the liver is the body's primary detoxification organ. Many chemicals cause disease and/or death as a result of direct toxicity to the liver. When this occurs, the injury is known medically as *hepatocellular necrosis*. The term necrosis is defined as cell death. If cells in the liver are destroyed at a rate faster than they can be reproduced, fatality will result. That is what happens when children are poisoned by household chemicals. It is what happens with poisonous berry or mushroom ingestion, and it is the same mechanism by which drug overdose kills. Drugs and many household chemicals may also damage the kidneys beyond repair. Additionally, the lungs are highly sensitive to damage by toxic substances, particularly those which liberate fumes such as bleach, solvents, lye, ammonia, paints and gasoline.

N-Acetyl cysteine is a variant of the amino acid cysteine. It is one of the most valuable aids for preventing the tissue damage resulting from exposure to or ingestion of toxic compounds. Currently, this compound is being used in medical centers around the world as an emergency treatment for poisoning.

NAC was first used in the treatment of a variety of chronic lung diseases, particularly those due to the accumulation of excess mucous. One of the effects of NAC is that it helps thin mucous. Thus, it is an excellent remedy for chronic lung diseases, sinus infections, colds, influenza and pneumonia.

Researchers have also found that NAC prevents lung damage induced by the inhalation of toxic chemical gases. Studies have shown that cellular damage is reduced by 50 percent or greater if NAC is taken during or shortly after the toxic exposure. In one study it was found that the toxicity due to noxious chemical inhalation impaired the functional capacity of the lung's immune cells. However, when NAC was added to the diet, their function rapidly returned to normal.

NAC is also highly protective for liver tissue. Studies have shown that, singlehandedly, it prevented life-threatening chemical-induced liver damage.

A partial list of the uses for NAC includes: 1) heavy metal detoxification---it is particularly active against mercury, silver and lead; 2) drug overdose; 3) toxic chemical exposure; 4) poisonous plant ingestion, including poisonous mushrooms; 5) bronchitis; 6) influenza; 7) pneumonia; 8) sinus infection; 9) ear infection.

In the event of a toxic exposure take three to four capsules of NAC every hour for 12 to 36 hours. To aid in the recovery after the toxic exposure three capsules taken four times daily should suffice. A similar dose would be effective for respiratory infections.

Chlorella

Chlorella is a single-cell fresh-water algae. It is a rich source of nutrients and contains more nutrition per pound than most commonly available foods.

The value of chlorella for survival is primarily a consequence of its nutritional content. One could live adequately on nothing but chlorella and water for several days. It is rich in amino acids, fatty acids and certain vitamins and minerals including B-12, beta carotene, iron and zinc. Chlorella is one of the few sources of B-12 in the vegetable kingdom. However, there is one substance in chlorella that supersedes all of these: nucleic acids. The nucleic acids are RNA and DNA: the genetic material. Chlorella is the richest known natural source of nucleic acids. These are crucial for the healing of wounds of all types and for increasing the body's resistance to stress.

Additionally, chlorella is the richest known source of chlorophyll. This unique substance has numerous beneficial functions. It helps support intestinal function, effectively preventing a variety of intestinal illnesses, including diarrhea, constipation, colitis, diverticulitis and ulcers. Studies have shown that it is extremely active in removing residues of toxic compounds, including hydrocarbons, pesticides, herbicides and heavy metals.

Chlorella exhibits a variety of pharmacological effects. Perhaps its greatest value is in chemical detoxification. If human exposure to toxic chemicals occurs, whether through the air (lungs), water or on the skin, the chemicals are readily absorbed into the internal system, gaining access to the blood and internal organs. This is where chlorella plays an important role. It binds toxic chemicals on contact, rendering them inactive and carries them out of the system through human wastes. Additionally, when toxic exposure occurs, chlorella helps repair the resultant damage to internal organs such as the liver, kidneys, intestines, pancreas and lungs.

Lastly, chlorella helps build strong blood. This is especially important when significant blood loss occurs. Its rich content of chlorophyll, B-12 and organically-bound iron assist in the formation of new, healthy red blood cells. The structure of chlorophyll is similar to that of hemoglobin, and this fact is one reason it is so useful in building new blood. In addition, chlorella's organically-bound iron is extremely well absorbed and readily assembled into the hemoglobin molecule. In is a superior and safer iron source than inorganic iron, the kind typically prescribed by doctors.

Chapter 7 Water Treatment and Accessories

In the event of a severe earthquake, potable water will be difficult to find. Potable water is defined as water that is safe to drink. In San Francisco, the tap water turned brown due to the breaking of water mains and its subsequent contamination with soil, dirt and sewage.

Contaminated drinking water is dangerous. If sewage lines are broken, that's when serious trouble begins. People who drink the water may rapidly develop life-threatening infections.

If bottled water is available, that would solve the problem. What if it isn't? Fortunately, a simple inexpensive method of water treatment has recently been developed. It is a water-treatment straw called *Clean Sip*. This straw is unique in that it utilizes three distinct methods of water treatment. The most valuable of these in terms of survival is a patented process called *electrochemical oxidation reduction.* In a nutshell, this process effectively destroys microbes by electroplating them against a special metallic medium. The result is that microbes are destroyed on contact.

Clean Sip also contains activated carbon which is invaluable for treating water tainted by noxious chemicals, since carbon effectively binds pesticides, herbicides, chlorine, heavy metals, hydrocarbons and hundreds of other compounds. The *Clean Sip* straw is ideal for the survival medicine kit. It is compact, and several can be easily stored in the car, at work or at home.

Acu-Filter is the name brand of an additional type of straw. It also helps prevent human intake of microbes. Additionally, this straw contains large quantities of activated carbon, making it the ideal one for removing toxic chemicals from the water.

Thus, if the water supply is contaminated by massive chemical or nuclear radiation leakages, *Acu-Filter* would be the straw of choice. In contrast, *Clean-Sip* is the preferable one for removing microbial contaminants. Both straws may be purchased by calling (800) 243-5242.

Water Treatment Units

In the scenario of a major earthquake, ready access to heating devices may be impossible. Even so, every attempt should be made to heat and preferably boil the water prior to consumption. An alternative approach would be to put the water into a clean, clear vessel, and place it in the sun for 12 hours. The sun's ultraviolet rays are highly toxic to microbes and can help sterilize water. The water concentrates the ultraviolet rays through a mechanism similar to a magnifying glass. This works best if the water is put into a glass container, since glass also magnifies the effects of solar rays.

The individual will be as prepared as is humanly possible for the worst if he/she are armed with effective water treatment devices. Remember, people in San Francisco, Santa Cruz and Watsonville, California lived with brown water for days. These Californians would have given anything to have had available an effective methods or systems for water treatment. The same happened in Armenia, Iran, Russia and, most recently, Turkey. A similar circumstance could happen anywhere in the world's earthquake and flood zones. It seems ironic that water, the essence of life, may also act as the potion of death.

Reliable water treatment units include pump-activated devices. These offer the benefit of being portable. Additionally, most have been tested and approved for effective removal of water-borne contaminants. Pump-activated devices can effectively remove chlorine after it is added to contaminated water. The addition of chlorine is a highly effective method for destroying microbes. However, because of the toxicity of chlorine, boiling is the preferred method of sterilization. The pump activated devices may be purchased in stores specializing in outdoor and sports equipment.

Possibly the simplest method for treating the water is to do what the municipalities do: add oxidizing agents to it. What they add is chlorine, and we could add that as well. However, as has been mentioned, chlorine is highly toxic and the slightest mishandling of it can result in burns and other serious illnesses.

Fortunately, a non-toxic oxidizing agent is available. Called *0-2-TheMax*, it is a special type of sodium chloride. It works by simply raising the pH to such a degree that large amounts of oxygen are liberated within the water. Oxygen is toxic to bacteria and, thus, the water is sterilized. Additionally, chlorite ions, which are a form of non-toxic chlorine, are released further ensuring sterilization. Within 10 minutes after application, the water should be potable. Still, advisable to boil the water and then add the sterilizing agents. In that manner, sterility is guaranteed.

Masks

The life-threatening danger of noxious gases was recently brought to public attention during the Gulf War. Gas mask companies sold hundreds of thousands of masks, and, even here in the United States, hundreds were sold largely as a consequence of nerve gas paranoia.

The use of masks could save lives in the event of toxic chemical or nuclear radiation releases. However, one need not don the cumbersome military-style masks used in the Gulf War. Specialized light-weight masks are now available. The North Safety Equipment Company offers numerous masks which are suitable for survival. They are light weight and easy to use. These masks effectively remove dust, petro-chemical fumes, acid gases, chlorine/bromine gases and all the gases produced by volatile hydrocarbons, which include kerosene, propane, natural gas, benzene and gasoline fumes. The North Company makes both disposable and reusable types of masks. The disposable type is ideal for emergency survival usage. The reusable type offers the advantage of the insertion of different types of cartridges. The additional cartridges required depend upon the type of chemical that is liberated. However, the standard unit will filter out and, thereby, prevent the inhalation of the most common noxious gases. The North mask may be ordered by calling *Nutritional Supplement Service*, (800) 243-5242.

Chapter 8 Conclusion

Natural disasters are an inevitable consequence of human existence. Societies have dealt with them for centuries. A few societies -- Pompeii, for one -- have been obliterated by them. Where and when they will strike can never be precisely predicted even by the most modern and advanced scientific tools.

Today, natural disasters happen worldwide on a daily basis. Despite this fact, most people have an indifferent attitude believing, in essence, "It couldn't happen to me." This way of thinking is particularly true of Americans. Yet, earthquakes regularly rock the Western states, tornadoes routinely shatter the Middle West, floods frequently smother the deep South and hurricanes seasonally batter the Eastern coastal states.

Major earthquakes occur throughout the world every year, and they affect millions. Over the last 15 years, well over a million people have been injured and nearly 500,000 killed by earthquakes. Thousands of others died as a consequence of diseases and injuries that occurred in the aftermath. Unfortunately, these latter deaths are rarely publicized. This means earthquakes claim more lives than any other type of natural disaster.

Should people in America be concerned about disasters of this scope? Is genocide in our country possible? Certainly, a toxic genocide is. In other words, it is more likely that disease and mass death will be the result of exposure to toxic chemicals or the release of nuclear radiation than from tidal waves, floods, earthquakes or the flow of molten lava. Yet, of all these dangers of Nature, the occurrence of a major earthquake in the United States sparks the greatest concerns for mass destruction. Additionally, in respect to the geology and climatology of the United States, it is the most probable of Nature's mass killers to strike us. However, while earthquakes concern only the segments of the population living along or near fault lines, toxic chemicals literally bathe us all.

Billions of gallons of toxic compounds are stored throughout the United States and Canada, and many millions of gallons are transported by rail and roadway every day. It cannot be disputed that if an earthquake is powerful enough, thousands of people could be killed instantly. Yet, in this highly industrialized society, hundreds of variables exist besides the brute force of Nature, variables which are not found in primitive societies. This makes the potential damage caused by earthquakes occurring in the Western world entirely unpredictable. For instance, in 1964 an earthquake measuring 8.3 on the Richter Scale struck Anchorage, Alaska. It was the strongest quake ever recorded on the continental U.S.A. One hundred and fifteen people were killed, which is considerable in such a sparsely populated state, and 75 percent of the state's industrial capacity was destroyed.

At the time of this writing earthquakes are rocking the earth, and volcanoes are erupting on a weekly basis throughout the Ring of Fire. Their rate of development is so pronounced that it is difficult for geologists and seismologists to keep up with the pace. For example, 250 earthquakes and aftershocks jarred Japan after recent (July, 1991) volcanic eruptions. Mount Pintatubo erupted in June, 1991, after 600 years of dormancy. Its eruptions decimated a huge U.S. Air Force base, rendering it inoperable. In the same year Hurricane Bob tore up much of the New England coast. In February/March of 1992 floods devastated much of Southern Texas. At one point nearly every interstate was under water. The powers of the environment appear to have gone haywire.

Other environmental disasters unrelated to the forces of

Nature are happening with frightening regularity. It seems that every month a major toxic spill or toxic substance release occurs somewhere in the U.S.A. In August of 1991 a spill of nuclear wastes occurred on a highway in Newport News, Virginia. Concern over toxicity was so great that a portion of the roadway was excavated. In September of 1991, two freight trains carrying hazardous materials collided head-on in Knott, Indiana. Tank cars carrying toxic compounds exploded, and massive toxic clouds were released. Everyone living within two miles of the accident site was evacuated. Numerous people were treated for symptoms of toxic gas inhalation. In November 1991, a freight train derailed and caught fire near Louisville, Kentucky. The derailment occurred over a railroad bridge, making it impossible for crisis workers to extinguish the flames. Fourteen tanker cars fell into the river. There was a great deal of concern, as one of the derailed tanker cars carried hydrogen cyanide, the most toxic, lethal gas known and the one responsible for the Bhopal massacre. An additional rail car was loaded with 74,000 pounds of cluster bombs. Fortunately, the fire was contained and a catastrophe avoided. Also in November of 1991, a tanker car containing sulfur dioxide exploded in Salt Lake City, Utah. Several hundred people were overcome by this noxious, highly irritating gas; dozens were hospitalized. The Oakland, California fire of October 1991, a bizarre catastrophe, destroyed 3,000 homes. Essentially, an entire district of that city was destroyed. Hundreds of people suffered from smoke inhalation, burns and minor wounds. Several people died. Perhaps of greatest concern is the recent rash of accidents at nuclear plants. For instance, in November of 1991, radioactive waste water was released from a nuclear plant in South Carolina. Over 50,000 gallons of radioactive water were "accidentally" spilled from holding tanks. This was followed by the release of radioactive steam. This is a major nuclear toxic incident, and, contrary to the party line, it will have a measurable, negative impact upon humans and the environment. What will happen next?

A great deal can be done to improve the readiness of the public, emotionally, psychologically and physically. The Survivor's Nutritional Pharmacy is a medicinal kit which employs only natural, non-toxic substances for the treatment of disaster-related conditions. All of the remedies mentioned in this booklet may be purchased from the Nutritional Supplement Services by calling (800) 243-5242. A complete summary of the various nutrients/remedies useful in the treatment of a number of survival related illnesses is found in Appendix A.

Natural remedies can be used to help prevent and/or treat illnesses. People with serious illnesses should always consult their physicians before applying any new therapy. However, in a survival setting, such consultations may be impossible. A nutritional pharmacy is the ideal solution, as its components will help in relieving some of the pain and in the prevention of agonizing illnesses. The remedies discussed in this booklet can help save lives, and with modern medicine that is always the bottom line.

Remember, a natural disaster could strike close to home at any time. Would you be ready if one were to happen right now?*

* Most of the predictions of this book recently came true (April 25th through 28th, 1992) after the latest USA earthquake occurring in Northern California. People living in the towns of Ferndale, Scotia and Petrolia in Northern California's Humbolt county know first hand the reality of these issues and how frightening it is to live in the world's earthquake zones, especially if ill-prepared: people without water, electricity, roofs over their heads, and threatened by all manner of toxic and environmental disasters, right here in the United States.

Appendix A

Virtually any type of illness could arise in the aftermath of a major environmental catastrophe. The following is a list of illnesses/diseases and injuries expected to occur under these circumstances along with the nutrients, medicines and herbs useful in their treatment:

Abrasions

Topical Treatment

Bee propolis
Tea tree oil
Aloe vera cream

Internal Treatment

Vitamin C
Vitamin E
Zinc

Asthma Attacks

Internal Treatment

Magnesium
Vitamin C
Pantothenic acid
Vitamin A
B-complex

Allergic Rashes

Topical Treatment

Tea tree oil
Sulfur drops or ointment
Vitamin C cream
Bee propolis ointment or spray
Aloe vera gel or cream

Internal Treatment

Vitamin C
Vitamin E
Aloe vera juice
Selenium
Bromelain

Anxiety Attack

Internal Treatment

Thiamine
Vitamin B-6
Magnesium
Tyrosine
Pantothenic acid
Calcium

Blood Clots

Internal Treatment

Bromelain
Vitamin E

Fish oils

Bruises

Topical Treatment

Bee propolis spray or ointment
Tea tree oil
Vitamin C cream

Internal Treatment

Bromelain
Vitamin E
Vitamin C
Bioflavonoids

Burns

Topical Treatment

Aloe
Sulfur drops/ointment
Bee propolis
Tea tree oil
Vitamin E oil

Internal Treatment

Vitamin E
Vitamin C
Pantothenic acid
Selenium
Zinc
Aloe vera juice

Note: The first step in the treatment of *chemical burns* is to flush the exposed site with copious amounts of water. Neutralization may be attempted if water is unobtainable. Use bicarbonate of soda to neutralize acid burns and vinegar to neutralize burns due to bases (i.e. lyes).

Cardiac Arrhythmia

Internal Treatment

Magnesium
Potassium
Thiamine
Coenzyme Q-10
Vitamin A drops
Pantothenic acid

Cuts/Lacerations/Puncture Wounds

Topical Treatment

Tea tree oil
Bee propolis
Liquid Trace Minerals
Sulfur drops

Internal Treatment

Vitamin C
Zinc
Pantothenic acid
Vitamin E
Vitamin A

Cold Sores

Topical Treatment

Tea tree oil
Bee propolis spray or ointment
Aloe vera gel or cream
Vitamin C cream
Vitamin E

Internal Treatment

Acidophilus
Aloe vera juice
Bee propolis capsules
Vitamin C
Bioflavonoids
Lateroflora
Lysine

Colitis

Internal Treatment

Chlorella
Aloe vera juice
Acidophilus
Pantothenic acid

Constipation

Internal Treatment

Chlorella
Aloe vera juice

Acidophilus
Magnesium
Pantothenic acid

Note: the number one cause of constipation is dehydration

Cystitis (Bladder Infection)

Internal Treatment

Cranberry concentrate
Chlorella
Vitamin A
Vitamin C
Garlic
Selenium
Acidophilus
Lateroflora

Diabetes (uncontrolled)

Internal Treatment

Chlorella
Selenium
Vitamin C
Niacinamide
Aloe vera juice
N-acetyl cysteine
Folic acid
Zinc
Vitamin B-6
Chromium

Diarrhea

Internal Treatment

Honey
Acidophilus
Folic acid
Aloe vera
Chlorella
Lateroflora

Eye Injuries

Topical Treatment

Aloe vera drops
Vitamin A drops

Internal Treatment

Vitamin A
Vitamin E
Vitamin C
Riboflavin
Folic acid
Zinc

Fractures or Severe Sprains

Topical Treatment

Vitamin C cream
Tea tree oil

Internal Treatment

Hydroxyapatite (MCHC)
Vitamin C
Vitamin A
Vitamin D
Magnesium
Multiple-mineral

Heat Exhaustion/Stroke

Topical Treatment

Aloe vera gel or liquid
Vitamin C cream

Internal Treatment

Pantothenic acid
Vitamin C
Aloe vera liquid
Potassium
Magnesium
Salt

Note: In heat exhaustion water should be consumed only when mixed with salt. Add 1/4 to 1/2 teaspoon of salt per 10 ounces of water. The salt is needed to enhance adrenal gland function.

Heavy Metal Poisoning

Internal Treatment

Selenium
Calcium

Magnesium
Zinc
Vitamin B-6
Niacin
Vitamin C
N-acetyl cysteine
Glutathione
Chlorella

Hepatitis

Internal Treatment

Beet Juice Flavonoid or tablets
Lipoic acid (known by the trade name *Thioctic*)
Liv-52
N-acetyl cysteine
Chlorella
Choline
Ginger root
Vitamin C
B-complex
Selenium
Dandelion root
Folic acid

Hypoglycemic Reaction

Internal Treatment

Chromium
Honey (or a similar source of natural sugar)
Chlorella
B-complex
Magnesium

Insecticide/Herbicide Poisoning

Topical Treatment

Aloe vera gel
Bee propolis spray
Sulfur drops

Internal Treatment

Selenium
Vitamin C
Vitamin B-6
Zinc
Garlic
Chlorella
N-acetyl cysteine
Glutathione

Toxic Chemical, Gas or Smoke Inhalation

Internal Treatment

Glutathione
Vitamin C
Beta carotene
Vitamin E
Folic acid
Selenium
Vitamin A
Zinc
N-acetyl cysteine

Radiation Exposure

Topical Treatment

Bee propolis spray
Aloe vera gel
Sulfur drops
Vitamin E

Internal Treatment

Beta carotene
Glutathione
N-acetyl cysteine
Selenium
Vitamin E
Vitamin C
Folic acid
Pantothenic acid
Chlorella
Garlic (aged or cooked)

Note: Research indicates that raw garlic is the least effective type for preventing radiation-induced damage. Aged garlic extract is preferable for use as an antioxidant.

Sinus Infection

Topical Treatment

Tea tree oil
Vitamin C cream

Internal Treatment

Vitamin A drops
Vitamin E
Vitamin C
B-complex
Chlorella
Garlic
Bromelain
Propolis

Sore Throats/Colds

Topical Treatment

Bee propolis spray
Tea tree oil (gargle/lozenge)
Honey

Internal Treatment

Vitamin C
Vitamin A
Garlic
Zinc
Bee Propolis (lozenges or capsules)
Honey
Acidophilus

Stomach or Duodenal Ulcers

Internal Treatment

Bee propolis
Pantothenic acid
Folic acid
Acidophilus

Aloe vera
Chlorella
Zinc

Tooth Ache or Gum Infection

Topical Treatment

Tea tree oil
Bee propolis (granules or spray)
Vitamin C cream

Internal Treatment

Vitamin C
Zinc
Acidophilus
Coenzyme Q-10

Toxic Chemical Ingestion

Internal Treatment

Chlorella
Vitamin C
Vitamin A
N-acetyl cysteine
Glutathione
Selenium
Vitamin E
Lipoic acid
Coenzyme Q-10

Vaginitis

Topical Treatment
Tea tree oil
Honey
Bee propolis spray
Vitamin E

Internal Treatment
Acidophilus
Selenium
Zinc
Garlic

Rabies

Topical Treatment
Raw garlic, crushed
Tea tree oil

Internal Treatment
Vitamin A
Bee propolis
Vitamin C
Acidophilus
Pycnogenol
Onion
Bioflavonoids
Folic acid
Pantothenic acid

Frostburn/Frostbite

Topical Treatment
Cayenne pepper ointment
Vitamin E

Internal Treatment
Cayenne pepper
Magnesium
Pycnogenol
Vitamin E
Vitamic C
Fish oils
Sardines
Garlic
Pantothenic acid

Ear Infections/Aches

Topical Treatment
Iodine (Lugol's Solution - 1 drop)

Internal Treatment
Zinc
Vitamin A
Vitamin C
Bee propolis
Garlic
Cayenne pepper
Pycnogenol

Appendix B

Symptoms Caused By Specific Diseases and Toxicities

The diagnosis of illnesses or diseases should be undertaken only by medically licensed practitioners. Americans are accustomed to the convenience of having access to the expertise of medical professionals at any hour of the day. If medical help is desired on Christmas day or New Year's eve, it can be gotten. Emergency rooms are almost never closed.

The survival setting presents that rare circumstance when medical professionals may be impossible to access, not just for hours but for days or even weeks. Therefore, it is imperative that the general public be made aware of the signs and symptoms of the various illnesses or diseases with which they might be confronted in the event of a natural or environmental disaster. In this section, only diseases which may be difficult to diagnose or which may be confused with other illness are included. The following is a list of these illnesses/diseases followed by the more commonly occurring signs and symptoms for each:

Arsenic Poisoning

Poisoning by arsenic is not as remote as it might seem. It is a component of various industrial chemicals as well as insecticides, fumigants, weed killers, fruit sprays and rat poisons. Arsene gas is highly toxic and is transported by truck and rail car. A certain number of deaths occur every year in the United States from environmental arsenic poisoning. Thousands of others are left chronically ill because of it. Symptoms of acute poisoning include:

skin lesions, dryness or excoriation
paralysis
confusion
headaches
muscular weakness
burning or tingling in limbs
petechiae (tiny skin hemorrhages)
nausea and vomiting
abdominal pain
loss of appetite
watery diarrhea (may be severe and persistent)

Congestive Heart Failure

This condition is most commonly seen in the elderly. It can be precipitated by stress and/or impaired nutrition. It is also common in individuals suffering from chronic lung disease.

fatigue, worsening upon exertion
swelling of the feet, ankles, face and/or eyelids
shortness of breath
cough
cold sweats
heart rhythm disturbances

Cyanide Poisoning

Cyanide is a highly toxic respiratory poison. It is fatal to man when consumed in amounts as low as 0.1 grams. Poisoning usually results from inhalation of hydrogen cyanide or hydrocyanic gas, although the ingestion of cyanide is also lethal. Cyanide compounds are rapidly absorbed and may cause death within minutes. Once inhaled, the gas is readily absorbed from the lungs into the bloodstream but may also be absorbed directly through the skin. Additionally, recent reports indicate that many fire-related deaths may be due to the inhalation of cyanide gas, which is liberated from burning building materials.

In the event of a massive release of cyanide gas, the logistics of self-protection are overwhelming. If this does occur, don a mask, protect the eyes, put on a rubber suit or rain suit, wear thick plastic or leather gloves, take megadoses of antioxidants and leave the region immediately. Signs and symptoms of cyanide poisoning include:

burning of the eyes and lungs
shortness of breath or respiratory distress
petechiae (small hemorrhages in the skin)
nausea and vomiting
almond-like odor from the breath and tissues
severe convulsions/seizures
severe abdominal pain and/or intestinal bleeding
cherry-red coloration of the skin
faintness and dizziness
sweating

Note: Acute cyanide poisoning usually results in death within 15 minutes and, thus, many of these symptoms are rarely seen.

Cystitis (Bladder Infection)

urinary urgency
pressure in the bladder
incomplete voiding
frequent urination
burning upon urination
pus or blood in the urine

pelvic or lower back pain

Hypoglycemic Reaction

fainting
shock
cold sweats
anxiety
agitation
irritability
anger or violent behavior
depression
sudden fatigue
delusions
headache
coma (usually occurs only in diabetics)

Hepatitis

yellow discoloration of the skin or whites of the eyes
nausea
loss of appetite
back or abdominal pain (right-sided)
weight loss (sudden)
diarrhea
maldigestion

Insecticide/Herbicide Poisoning (acute)

respiratory distress
loss of appetite
nausea and vomiting
muscle weakness

numbness (loss of sensation)
twitching
tremors
muscle cramps or twitching
rapid heart beat
muscular paralysis
loss of coordination
paralysis
coma

Mercury Poisoning

Mercury poisoning can occur in several ways besides touching or swallowing globs of mercury. This highly toxic metal is used in the manufacture of a variety of chemicals, and millions of pounds of it are found in storage tanks and/or are transported in the form of solid, liquid and gaseous compounds every year.

Certain industrial chemicals, as well as numerous insecticides and fungicides, contain mercury. Thus, a possibility exists that the spillage or explosion of a tanker car or truckload of mercury or compounds containing it could cause an environmental disaster of the most extreme kind.

Mercurial compounds are potent destroyers of human protein. Therefore, they inactivate the most crucial proteins for survival: the enzymes. In addition, mercury binds to cell membrane proteins, leading to the rupture of cells and, therefore, their death. Toxicity may occur through inhalation, skin contact or ingestion. Symptoms of acute poisoning include:

diarrhea
abdominal pain
respiratory distress

loss of sensation
loss of coordination
headache

Myocardial Infarction (Heart Attack)

This often fatal occurrence typically begins with severe chest pain, usually left-sided, radiating to any of the following areas:

the neck
the shoulders
the throat
the left arm (most commonly)
the right arm (rarely)
the jaw

Other symptoms include:

nausea
heartburn
cold sweats
coldness of the body
fatigue and/or sleepiness
apathy

Peptic Ulcer (Stomach or Duodenal Ulcer)

abdominal pain often relieved by eating
abdominal cramping
blood in the stool (dark red or black)
vomiting of blood
nausea and/or vomiting
diarrhea

Pneumonia

cough, usually productive
fever, usually above 101 degrees
chills
cold or hot sweats
fatigue, worse upon exertion
muscular pain and/or weakness
loss of appetite
shortness of breath more noticeable with exertion

Pyelonephritis (Kidney Infection)

Symptoms are the same as with bladder infection, plus:
lower back pain (not as low in the back as cystitis)

flank pain
chills and/or fever
cold sweats
high temperature
swollen eyelids or swelling beneath the eyes

Radiation Poisoning

nausea and vomiting
headache
fatigue
loss of appetite
diarrhea (may be severe)
hemorrhaging (from the mouth, rectum or vagina)
skin hemorrhages
weight loss
hair loss

dry skin and/or excoriation of the skin
metallic taste

Note: The symptom of metallic taste is characteristic of direct exposure to radioactive chemicals via inhalation.

Appendix C

Ordering Information for Nutritional Products, Books, Tapes and Survival Aids

All products listed may be ordered by contacting:

Nutritional Supplement Service
212 Willow Parkway
Buffalo Grove, Illinois 60089
Phone: (800) 243-5242

Note: This toll-free number is for orders only

Books

Books may be purchased by the public in bulk. Discounts are as follows:

1-5 books:	Retail plus $3.75 shipping and handling
6-12 books:	Less 10% plus $4.95 shipping and handling
13-24 books:	Less 15% plus $6.95 shipping and handling
25-83 books:	Less 20% plus $12.95 shipping and handling
84-167 books:	Less 30% - Call for shipping and handling
168 or more:	Less 25% plus $20.00 shipping and handling

Iowa, Illinois, and California residents must add sales tax.

Discounts for retailers are available. For more information call (800) 243-5242.

Tapes

Dr. Igram has produced in his professional studios a 3-tape set of audio cassettes on survival medicine for natural disasters. The tapes cover natural therapies and additional information not listed in the book, which is primarily for counteracting the following:

- nuclear radiation leakage
- toxic chemical releases/spills
- wounds and other traumatic injuries
- burns
- water-borne illnesses
- diseases due to stress and/or exposure
- infectious diseases

To order send $34.95 plus $5.00 shipping and handling to:

A.I.C.M.
212 Willow Parkway
Buffalo Grove, Illinois 60089

To place credit card orders for books or tapes call:

(800) 243-5242

Bibliography

Abraham, A.S., et al. 1987. Magnesium in the prevention of lethal arrhythmias in acute myocardial infarction. *Arch. Intern. Med.*a 147:753

American Red Cross. 1973. *Standard First Aid and Personal Safety*. New York: Double Day, Inc.

Barry, B.E., Miller. F.J., and J.D. Crapo. 1982. Alveolar epithelial injury caused by inhalation of .25 ppm of ozone. In Lee, S.D., et al (ed). *The Biomedical Effects of Ozone and Related Photochemical Oxidants*. Proceedings of an International Symposium. Princeton, NJ: Scientific Publishers.

Bekiarova, G.I., Markova, M.P., and V.G. Kagan. 1989. Alpha-Tocopherol protection of erythrocytes from hemolysis induced by thermal injury. *Bull. Eksp. Biol. Med.* 107:413.

Belalche, P. 1985. Treatment of skin infections with the essential oil of Melaleuca alternifolia. *Phytotherapie* 15:15-17.

Belalche, P. 1985. Treatment of vaginal infections of Candida albicans with the essential oil of Melaleuca alternifolia. *Ibid*, p. 13-15.

Binkova, B., et al. 1988. Damage and repair of human lymphocyte DNA under the activation of molecular oxygen. *Bull. Eksp. Biol. Med.* 106:676.

Boyd, M.R., et al. 1982. Protective role of endogenous pulmonary glutathione conjugates with the microsomally activated pulmonary bronchiolar alkylating agent and cytotoxin, 4 ipomeanol. *J. Pharm. Exp. Ther.* 215:97.

Brodribb, A.J.M., and C.R. Rickets. 1971. The effect of zinc in the healing of burns. *Injury* 3:25.

Brown, M.H. 1987. *The Toxic Cloud.* New York: Perennial Library, Harper & Row.

Bucci, L.R. 1988. Proteolytic enzymes and acute injuries. *Chir. Prod.* June, p. 52-55.

Bunta, S., and B. Prodrumac. 1978. Anti-inflammatory Effect of Propolis. *Apimondia International Symposium on Apitherapy*, Portoroz, Yugoslavia, Sept.

Burch, G.E., and T.D. Giles. 1977. The importance of magnesium deficiency in cardiovascular disease. *Amer. Heart J.* 94:649-57

Carson, D.A., Seto, S. and D. B. Watson. 1986. Lymphocyte dysfunction after DNA damage by toxic oxygen species. *J. Exp. Med.* 163:746-51.

Chasseaud, L.F. 1979. The role of glutathione and glutathione S-transferases in the metabolism of chemical carcinogens and other electrophilic agents. *Adv. Cancer Res.* 29:175-275.

Chatterjee, I.B. 1978. Ascorbic acid metabolism. *World. Rev. Nutr. Diet* 30:669-87.

Chernov, M.S., et al. 1971. Prevention of stress ulcers. *Amer. J. Surg.* 122:674.

Chernov, M.S.1972. Stress ulcer: a preventable disease. *J. Trauma* 12:831.

Cirelli, M.G. 1967. Five years of clinical experience with bromelains in therapy of edema and inflammation in postoperative tissue reaction, skin infections and trauma. *Clin. Med.* 74:55-59.

Coats, Bill C. 1979. *The Silent Healer: A Modern Study of Aloe*. Garland, Texas: Coats.

Cody, V., et al. (eds). 1986. *Plant Flavonoids in Biology and Medicine*. New York: A.R. Liss.

Collip, P.J., et al. 1975. Pyridoxine treatment of childhood bronchial asthma. *Ann. Allergy* 35:93.

Cragin, R.B. 1962. The use of bioflavonoids in the prevention and treatment of athletic injuries. *Med. Times* 90:529.

DeFlora, S., et al. 1985. In. The effects of N-acetylcysteine on glutathione metabolism and the biotransformation of carcinogens and/or toxic compounds. *Carcinogenesis* 6:1735-45.

Diplock, A.T. 1981. The role of vitamin E and selenium in the prevention of oxygen-induced tissue damage. In. *Selenium in Biology and Medicine, Proceedings Second International Symposium,* 1980. Westport, CT: AVI Publishing.

Danhof, I.E., and B.H. McAnally. 1983. Stabilized aloe vera: Effect on human skin cells. *Drug Cosmet. Ind.* 133:52.

Ershoff, B.H. 1952. Effects of vitamin A malnutriture on resistance to stress. *Proc. Soc. Exp. Biol. Med.* 79:580.

Felton, G.E. 1981. Fibrinolytic and antithrombotic action of bromelain may eliminate thrombosis in heart patients. *Med. Hypothesis* 6:99.

Forman, H.J., et al. 1983. Role of selenium and sulfur-containing amino acids protection against oxygen toxicity. *Lab. Invest.*

Frolkis, V.V., et al. 1987. Antioxidants as antiarrhythmic drugs. *Cardiology* 74:124.

Fromer, D.J. 1975. The healing of gastric ulcers by zinc sulfate. *Med. J. Aust.* 2:793.

Fusi, S., et al. 1984. Reversal of post-burn immunosuppression by the administration of vitamin A. *Surgery* 96:330.

Gabor, M. 1972. Pharmacologic effect of flavonoids on blood vessels. *Angiologica* 9:355.

Gage, Diane. 1988. *Aloe Vera*. Rochester, Vermont: Healing Arts Press.

Gerber, L.E., and J.W. Erdman, Jr. 1981. Wound healing in rats fed small supplements of retinyl acetate, beta carotene or retinoic acid. *Fed. Proc.* March 1, p.838.

Gerchman, R., et al. 1954. Oxygen poisoning and x-irradiation: a mechanism in common. *Science* 119:623-26.

Gilliland, S.E., and M.K. Speck. 1977. Antagonistic action of Lactobacillus acidophilus toward intestinal and food borne pathogens in associative cultures. *J. Food Product.* 40:830.

Gloor, M., and H. Fischer. 1971. Principles of flavonoid therapy. *Fortschr. Med.* 89:1025.

Green, H.N., and E. Mellanby. 1928. Vitamin A as an anti-infective agent. *Br. Med. J.* 20:691.

Gould, J.M., and B.A. Goldman. 1990. *Deadly Deceit: Low Level Radiation High Level Cover-Up*. New York: Four Walls Eight Windows.

Hagen, T.M., et al. 1990. Bioavailability of dietary glutathione: effect on plasma concentration. *American Physiological Society*,
G524.

Haley, J.V. 1979. Zinc sulfate and wound healing. *J. Surg. Res.*
27:168.

Heggers, J.P., et al. 1979. Dermaide aloe/aloe vera gel: comparison of the anti-microbial effects. *J. Amer. Med. Tech.* 41:293.

Hill, R. 1977. *Propalis--The Natural Antibiotic*. England: Thorsons Publishers Limited.

Humphrey, E. 1930. A new Australian germicide. *Med. J. Australia* January, p. 417.

Hunt, T.K., et al. 1969. Effect of vitamin A on reversing the inhibitory effect of cortisone on healing of open wounds in animals and man. *Ann. Surg.* 181:836.

Igram, Cass. 1989. *Eat Right or Die Young*. Cedar Rapids, IA: Literary Visions Publishing, Inc.
3
Iseri, L.T., et al. 1975. Magnesium deficiency and cardiac disorders. *Amer. J. Med.* 58:837.

Ishiyama, T., et al. 1976. A clinical study of the effect of coenzyme Q on congestive heart failure. *Japan Heart. J.* 17:32.

Ito, C., et al. 1979. Anti-inflammatory actions of proteases, bromelain, trypsin and their mixed preparations. *Folia Pharmachol. Japan* 75:227.

Jacobson, J.M., et al. 1990. *J. Appl. Physiol.* 68:1252-59.

Ketterer, B., Coles, B., and D.J. Meyer. 1983. The role of glutathione in detoxification. *Envir. Hlth Perspec.* 49:59.

Kucher, A.G. 1966. On the use of vitamins P and C for the prevention of increased capillary fragility in children. *Vopr. Pitan.* 25:39.

Lash, L.H., Hagen, T.M., and D.P. Jones. 1986. Exogenous glutathione protects intestinal epithelial cells from oxidative injury. *Proc. Natl. Acad. Sci.* 83:4641.

Lecomte, J., and H. Van Cauwenberge. 1971. Pharmacologic properties of bioflavonoids. *Rev. Med. Liege.* 26:673-81.

Leonart, M.S.S. 1989. Effect of vitamin E on red blood cell preservation. *Braz. J. Med. Biol. Res.* 22:85-6.

Levine, S.A., and P.M. Kidd. 1985. *Antioxidant Adaptation: Its Role in Free Radical Pathology*. San Leandro, CA: Allergy Research Group.

London, J., and J.O. Gibson. 1988. Pharmaceuticals containing terpenes and vitamin E for the treatment of cuts, burns, and abrasions. US 4,784,842. Nov. 15, 4 pp.

Lorber, A., et al. 1973. Clinical application for heavy metal-complexing potential of N-acetylcysteine. *J. Clin. Pharmacol.* 13:332.

Mathieson, P.W., Willliams, G. and J.E. MacSweeney. 1985. Survival after massive ingestion of carbon tetrachloride treated by intravenous acetylcysteine. *Human Toxicology* 4:627-31.

Menzel, D.B. 1979. Nutritional needs in environmental intoxication: vitamin E and air pollution, an example. *Env. Health Perspec.* 29:105.

Mills, T.J., et al. 1965. The use of a whole bone extract in the treatment of fractures. *Manitoba Medical Review* 45:92-6.

Milton, R.C. 1987. Mild vitamin A deficiency and childhood morbidity---an Indian experience. *Amer. J. Clin. Nutr.* 46:827.

Munan, L.P., and A. Einbeber. 1951. Calcium pantothenate and burns. *Br. Med. J.* Nov. 17, p. 1224.

Pan, G.D., and A. Huitson. 1987. Oral Fabrol (N-acetylcysteine) in chronic bronchitis. *Eur. Resp. J.* 1:351.

Paris, R., and J. Moury. 1964. Effects of diverse flavonoids upon capillary permeability. *Ann. Pharm. Frac.* 22:489-93.

Passwater, R. 1980. *Selenium as a Food and Medicine.* New Canaan, Conn: Keat's Publishing.

Pena, E. 1962. Melaleuca alternifolia oil: its use for trichomonal vaginitis and other vaginal infections. *Obstetrics and Gynecology* 19:793-5.

Pensfold, A. 1937. Some notes on the essential oil of Melaleuca alternifolia. *Australian J. Pharm.* March p. 274.

Rakesh, K., et al. 1987. Glutathione, a first line of defense against cadmium toxicity. *FASEB J.* 1:220-23.

Rasmussen, J.B., and C. Glennow. 1988. Reduction in days of illness after long-term treatment with N-acetylcysteine controlled-release tablets in patient with chronic bronchitis. *Eur. Resp. J.* 1:351:55.

Richardson, S. 1990. Aromas for asthmatics. *M.D.* Feb 14.

Robins, S.L., and R. S. Cotran. 1979. *Pathologic Basis of Disease.* Philadelphia, PA: W.B. Saunders.

Rodriguez-Bigas, M., Cruz, N.I., and A. Suarez. 1988. Comparative evaluation of aloe vera in the management of burn wounds in guinea pigs. Plastic and Reconstruct. *Surg.* 81:386.

Shahani, K.M., et al. 1977. *Cultured Dairy Products Journal* 12:8.

Shahani, K.M., and A.D. Ayebo. 1980. Role of dietary lactobacilli in gastrointestinal microecology. *Amer. J. Clin. Nutr.* 33:2448-2457.

Sommer, A. 1990. Vitamin A status, resistance to infection, and childhood mortality. *Ann. NY Acad. Sci.* 587:17.

Tseng, S.C.G., et al. 1985. Topical retinoid treatment for various dry eye disorders. *Ophthalmology*.

Uhlig, G., and J. Seifert. 1981. Efficacy of proteolytic enzymes traumanase (bromelain) on post traumatic edema. *Forsch. Med.* 99:554-56.

Urano, S. 1989. Stabilizing effect of vitamin E. *Bitamin* 63:75.

Vincent, J.G., Veomett, R.C., and R.F. Riley. 1959. Antibacterial activity associated with Lactobacillus acidophilus. *J. Bacteriol.* 78:477.

Wagner, P.D., et al. 1989. Protection against pulmonary O_2 toxicity by N-acetylcysteine. *Eur. Resp. J.* 2:116.

Walker, M. 1972. Clinical investigation of Australian Melaleuca alternifolia oil for a variety of common foot problems. *Current Podiatry* April.

Wolf, H. and W. Seeger. 1981. Prevention of respiratory distress syndrome by high dose alpha-tocopherol: experimental results and clinical aspects. Int. *J. Vit. Nutr. Res.* 51:181-83.

Wright, J. 1984. *Survive: The Earthquake Awaits.* CA: J.Wright